*Welcome to the **"Cookbook for Seniors: 110+ Recipes for Senior Adults Living with Chronic Kidney Disease."** This cookbook is designed to be a comprehensive resource for seniors navigating the complexities of managing chronic kidney disease (CKD) through delicious and nutritious cooking.*

Chronic kidney disease can present unique challenges for seniors, impacting not only their physical health but also their overall well-being and quality of life. From managing dietary restrictions to ensuring adequate nutrition, the journey with CKD requires careful attention to every meal. That's where this cookbook comes in.

In these pages, you will find a treasure trove of 110+ recipes specifically tailored to support seniors living with chronic kidney disease. Each recipe is crafted with the nutritional needs of seniors in mind, focusing on ingredients that promote kidney health while still tantalizing the taste buds.

We understand that cooking for CKD can seem daunting, but it doesn't have to be. Whether you're a seasoned home cook or just starting out in the kitchen, the recipes in this cookbook are designed to be accessible, easy to follow, and, most importantly, delicious.

Throughout the book, you'll find a diverse array of recipes spanning breakfast, lunch, dinner, and snacks, ensuring that every meal is a satisfying and nourishing experience. From comforting soups and hearty stews to vibrant salads and flavorful main courses, there's something for every palate and preference.

But this cookbook is more than just a collection of recipes. It's a guide to better health and wellness for seniors living with CKD. Each recipe is accompanied by helpful tips and nutritional information, empowering seniors to make informed choices about their diet and lifestyle.

We believe that good food has the power to heal and nourish, and that's why we've poured our hearts into creating this cookbook. Whether you're cooking for yourself or a loved one, we hope these recipes bring joy, comfort, and vitality to your table.

So grab your apron, sharpen your knives, and let's embark on a culinary journey toward better kidney health and overall wellness. Here's to good food, good health, and good living for seniors with chronic kidney disease.

1. Oatmeal with blueberries and honey

Ingredients:
- 1 cup old-fashioned oats
- 2 cups unsweetened almond milk (or low-fat milk)
- 1/2 cup fresh or frozen blueberries
- 1-2 tbsp honey (or to taste)

Instructions:

1. In a medium saucepan, bring the almond milk (or low-fat milk) to a simmer over medium heat.

2. Add the oats and cook, stirring occasionally, for 5-7 minutes until the oats are tender and the mixture has thickened.

3. Remove from heat and stir in the blueberries and honey.

4. Serve warm.

This recipe is a good option for seniors with chronic kidney disease for a few reasons:

- Oats are a whole grain that is low in phosphorus, which is important for managing kidney disease.

- Blueberries are a low-potassium fruit, which is also important for kidney-friendly diets.

- Honey provides natural sweetness without added sugars, which can be beneficial for managing blood sugar levels.

- Almond milk or low-fat milk are lower in phosphorus compared to regular milk.

Be sure to consult with a registered dietitian or healthcare provider to ensure this recipe fits within your specific dietary needs for chronic kidney disease.

2. Rice cereal with almond milk

Ingredients:
- 1 cup unsweetened rice cereal
- 1 cup unsweetened almond milk
- 1-2 tsp honey (optional)

Instructions:

1. In a bowl, combine the rice cereal and almond milk.

2. Microwave for 1-2 minutes, stirring halfway, until the cereal is warm and the milk is slightly thickened.

3. If desired, stir in 1-2 tsp of honey to add a touch of sweetness.

4. Serve warm.

This recipe is a good option for seniors with chronic kidney disease for a few reasons:

- Rice cereal is low in phosphorus, which is important for managing kidney disease.

- Almond milk is lower in phosphorus and potassium compared to regular dairy milk, making it a better choice.

- Honey provides natural sweetness without added sugars, which can be beneficial for managing blood sugar levels.

Be sure to choose an unsweetened rice cereal and unsweetened almond milk to keep the phosphorus and potassium content low. You can also adjust the amount of honey to your taste preferences.

As always, it's important to consult with a registered dietitian or healthcare provider to ensure this recipe fits within your specific dietary needs for chronic kidney disease.

3. Scrambled egg whites with bell peppers

Ingredients:
- 4 large egg whites
- 1/4 cup diced bell pepper (any color)
- 1 tbsp unsweetened almond milk
- 1/4 tsp garlic powder
- Salt and pepper to taste

Instructions:
1. In a small bowl, whisk together the egg whites, almond milk, garlic powder, salt, and pepper.

2. Spray a non-stick skillet with cooking spray and heat over medium heat.

3. Add the diced bell pepper and sauté for 2-3 minutes until slightly softened.

4. Pour the egg white mixture into the skillet and use a spatula to gently scramble the eggs, stirring frequently, until they are cooked through, about 3-5 minutes.

5. Serve hot.

This recipe is a good option for seniors with chronic kidney disease for a few reasons:

- Egg whites are a high-quality protein source that is low in phosphorus, which is important for managing kidney disease.

- Bell peppers are a low-potassium vegetable, making them a good choice for kidney-friendly diets.

- Almond milk is lower in phosphorus and potassium compared to regular dairy milk.

- The recipe is simple and easy to prepare, which can be beneficial for seniors who may have limited mobility or energy.

Be sure to avoid adding any cheese or other high-phosphorus ingredients to this dish. You can also adjust the amount of salt and pepper to your taste preferences.

As always, it's important to consult with a registered dietitian or healthcare provider to ensure this recipe fits within your specific dietary needs for chronic kidney disease.

4. Apple cinnamon quinoa

Ingredients:
- 1 cup uncooked quinoa, rinsed
- 2 cups unsweetened almond milk
- 1 medium apple, peeled, cored, and diced
- 1 tsp ground cinnamon
- 1-2 tbsp honey (optional)

Instructions:

1. In a medium saucepan, combine the rinsed quinoa and almond milk. Bring to a boil over high heat.

2. Once boiling, reduce heat to low, cover, and simmer for 15-20 minutes, or until the quinoa is tender and the liquid is absorbed.

3. Remove from heat and stir in the diced apple and cinnamon.

4. If desired, drizzle with 1-2 tablespoons of honey for added sweetness.

5. Serve warm.

This recipe is a good option for seniors with chronic kidney disease for a few reasons:

- Quinoa is a whole grain that is low in phosphorus, which is important for managing kidney disease.

- Apples are a low-potassium fruit, making them a good choice for kidney-friendly diets.

- Cinnamon adds flavor without the need for additional salt or sugar.

- Almond milk is lower in phosphorus and potassium compared to regular dairy milk.

- The recipe is easy to prepare and can be a nutritious breakfast or snack.

Be sure to use unsweetened almond milk and adjust the amount of honey to your taste preferences. You can also try other low-potassium fruits like berries or pears in place of the apple.

As always, it's important to consult with a registered dietitian or healthcare provider to ensure this recipe fits within your specific dietary needs for chronic kidney disease.

5. Low-sodium whole wheat toast with unsalted butter

Ingredients:
- 2 slices of low-sodium whole wheat bread
- 1-2 tsp unsalted butter

Instructions:
1. Toast the whole wheat bread slices until lightly golden brown.

2. Spread 1-2 tsp of unsalted butter evenly over the toast slices.

3. Serve immediately.

This recipe is a good option for seniors with chronic kidney disease for a few reasons:

- Whole wheat bread is a good source of fiber and is lower in phosphorus compared to white bread.

- Using unsalted butter helps to keep the sodium content low, which is important for managing kidney disease.

- The combination of whole grains and healthy fats from the butter can provide a satisfying and nutritious snack or light meal.

Some additional tips:

- Look for whole wheat bread that is labeled "low-sodium" or contains less than 140mg of sodium per slice.

- You can also try using a plant-based, unsalted butter alternative if preferred.

- Avoid adding any additional toppings or seasonings that may be high in sodium.

As always, it's important to consult with a registered dietitian or healthcare provider to ensure this recipe fits within your specific dietary needs for chronic kidney disease. They can provide personalized guidance on appropriate portion sizes and other dietary considerations.

6. Rice pancakes with fresh berries

Ingredients:
- 1 cup cooked white rice, cooled
- 2 large eggs
- 2 tbsp unsweetened almond milk
- 1 tsp vanilla extract
- 1/4 tsp ground cinnamon
- 1 cup fresh berries (such as blueberries, raspberries, or blackberries)
- Unsalted butter or non-stick cooking spray for cooking

Instructions:

1. In a medium bowl, mash the cooked rice with a fork until it forms a smooth, spreadable consistency.

2. Add the eggs, almond milk, vanilla, and cinnamon to the rice and mix well until fully combined.

3. Heat a non-stick skillet or griddle over medium heat and lightly grease with unsalted butter or non-stick cooking spray.

4. Scoop 1/4 cup portions of the rice batter onto the hot surface and cook for 2-3 minutes per side, or until golden brown.

5. Serve the rice pancakes warm, topped with fresh berries.

This recipe is a good option for seniors with chronic kidney disease for a few reasons:

- White rice is low in phosphorus, making it a kidney-friendly grain choice.

- Eggs provide high-quality protein without excessive phosphorus.

- Almond milk is lower in phosphorus and potassium compared to regular dairy milk.

- Fresh berries are a low-potassium fruit option.

- The recipe is simple to prepare and can be a nutritious breakfast or snack.

Be sure to avoid any high-sodium or high-phosphorus toppings or syrups. You can also experiment with other low-potassium fruit options, such as sliced peaches or kiwi.

As always, consult with a registered dietitian or healthcare provider to ensure this recipe fits within your specific dietary needs for chronic kidney disease.

7. Smoothie with almond milk, spinach, and berries

Ingredients:
- 1 cup unsweetened almond milk
- 1 cup fresh spinach leaves
- 1 cup frozen mixed berries (such as blueberries, raspberries, and blackberries)
- 1 tbsp honey (optional)

Instructions:
1. Add the almond milk, spinach, and frozen berries to a high-powered blender.

2. Blend on high speed until the mixture is smooth and creamy, about 1-2 minutes.

3. If desired, add 1 tbsp of honey and blend again briefly to incorporate.

4. Pour the smoothie into a glass and enjoy immediately.

This smoothie recipe is a good option for seniors with chronic kidney disease for several reasons:

- Almond milk is lower in phosphorus and potassium compared to regular dairy milk, making it a better choice.

- Spinach is a nutrient-dense green that is low in potassium, an important consideration for kidney health.

- Berries are a low-potassium fruit option that provide antioxidants and fiber.

- Honey can add natural sweetness without the need for added sugars.

The combination of the almond milk, spinach, and berries creates a nutrient-rich, kidney-friendly smoothie that can be a refreshing and satisfying snack or light meal.

As always, it's important to consult with a registered dietitian or healthcare provider to ensure this smoothie recipe fits within your specific dietary needs for chronic kidney disease. They can provide guidance on appropriate portion sizes and any other dietary considerations.

8. Greek yogurt with honey and strawberries

Ingredients:
- 1 cup plain, unsweetened Greek yogurt
- 1-2 tbsp honey
- 1 cup fresh strawberries, sliced

Instructions:
1. In a bowl, spoon the Greek yogurt.

2. Drizzle 1-2 tablespoons of honey over the yogurt, to taste.

3. Top with the sliced fresh strawberries.

4. Serve chilled.

This recipe is a good option for seniors with chronic kidney disease for a few reasons:

- Greek yogurt is a good source of protein without excessive phosphorus, which is important for managing kidney disease.

- Honey provides natural sweetness without added sugars, which can be beneficial for managing blood sugar levels.

- Strawberries are a low-potassium fruit option.

Some additional tips:

- Choose a plain, unsweetened Greek yogurt to keep the phosphorus and potassium content low.

- Adjust the amount of honey to your taste preferences.

- You can also try other low-potassium fruit options, such as blueberries or raspberries, in place of the strawberries.

As always, it's important to consult with a registered dietitian or healthcare provider to ensure this recipe fits within your specific dietary needs for chronic kidney disease. They can provide personalized guidance on appropriate portion sizes and other dietary considerations.

9. Cottage cheese with peaches

Ingredients:
- 1 cup low-fat cottage cheese
- 1 medium peach, sliced
- 1-2 tsp honey (optional)

Instructions:
1. In a bowl, spoon the cottage cheese.

2. Top the cottage cheese with the sliced peach.

3. If desired, drizzle 1-2 teaspoons of honey over the top.

4. Serve chilled.

This recipe is a good option for seniors with chronic kidney disease for a few reasons:

- Cottage cheese is a good source of protein without excessive phosphorus, which is important for managing kidney disease.

- Peaches are a low-potassium fruit option.

- Honey provides natural sweetness without added sugars, which can be beneficial for managing blood sugar levels.

Some additional tips:

- Choose a low-fat or reduced-fat cottage cheese to keep the phosphorus and sodium content lower.

- Adjust the amount of honey to your taste preferences, or omit it entirely if desired.

- You can also try other low-potassium fruit options, such as berries or pears, in place of the peaches.

As always, it's important to consult with a registered dietitian or healthcare provider to ensure this recipe fits within your specific dietary needs for chronic kidney disease. They can provide personalized guidance on appropriate portion sizes and other dietary considerations.

10. Low-sodium bagel with cream cheese

Ingredients:
- 1 low-sodium whole wheat bagel
- 2 tbsp low-fat or reduced-fat cream cheese

Instructions:

1. Toast the low-sodium whole wheat bagel until lightly golden brown.

2. Spread 2 tablespoons of low-fat or reduced-fat cream cheese evenly over the toasted bagel.

3. Serve immediately.

This recipe is a good option for seniors with chronic kidney disease for a few reasons:

- Low-sodium whole wheat bagels are lower in phosphorus and sodium compared to regular bagels, making them a better choice for kidney-friendly diets.

- Cream cheese is a good source of protein without excessive phosphorus.

- The combination of the whole grain bagel and protein-rich cream cheese can provide a satisfying and nutritious snack or light meal.

Some additional tips:

- Look for whole wheat bagels that are specifically labeled as "low-sodium" or contain less than 140mg of sodium per serving.

- Choose a low-fat or reduced-fat cream cheese to keep the saturated fat and calorie content lower.

- Avoid adding any additional toppings or seasonings that may be high in sodium.

As always, it's important to consult with a registered dietitian or healthcare provider to ensure this recipe fits within your specific dietary needs for chronic kidney disease. They can provide personalized guidance on appropriate portion sizes and other dietary considerations.

11. Cucumber and dill salad

Ingredients:
- 2 medium cucumbers, sliced
- 2 tbsp fresh dill, chopped
- 1 tbsp white wine vinegar
- 1 tsp olive oil
- Salt and pepper to taste

Instructions:

1. In a medium bowl, combine the sliced cucumbers and chopped fresh dill.

2. Drizzle the white wine vinegar and olive oil over the cucumbers and dill. Toss gently to coat.

3. Season with a small amount of salt and pepper to taste.

4. Chill the salad in the refrigerator for at least 30 minutes before serving to allow the flavors to meld.

This recipe is a good option for seniors with chronic kidney disease for a few reasons:

- Cucumbers are a low-potassium vegetable, making them a good choice for kidney-friendly diets.

- Fresh dill adds flavor without the need for high-sodium seasonings.

- The vinegar and olive oil provide a light, refreshing dressing without added sodium or phosphorus.

- The salad is easy to prepare and can be a cooling, hydrating side dish or snack.

Some additional tips:

- Use a small amount of salt, as needed, to avoid excessive sodium intake.

- You can also try adding a small amount of lemon juice or white wine vinegar for extra flavor.

- Adjust the amounts of the ingredients to suit your taste preferences.

As always, it's important to consult with a registered dietitian or healthcare provider to ensure this recipe fits within your specific dietary needs for chronic kidney disease.

12. Apple and walnut salad

Ingredients:
- 2 medium apples, cored and diced
- 1/4 cup chopped walnuts
- 2 tbsp plain, unsweetened Greek yogurt
- 1 tbsp lemon juice
- 1 tsp honey (optional)
- Ground cinnamon (optional)

Instructions:
1. In a medium bowl, combine the diced apples and chopped walnuts.

2. In a small bowl, mix together the Greek yogurt, lemon juice, and honey (if using).

3. Pour the yogurt dressing over the apple and walnut mixture and toss gently to coat.

4. Sprinkle a small amount of ground cinnamon over the top, if desired.

5. Chill the salad in the refrigerator for at least 30 minutes before serving.

This recipe is a good option for seniors with chronic kidney disease for a few reasons:

- Apples are a low-potassium fruit option.

- Walnuts provide a source of healthy fats without excessive phosphorus.

- Greek yogurt is a good source of protein without too much phosphorus.

- Lemon juice and cinnamon add flavor without the need for high-sodium seasonings.

Some additional tips:

- Choose a plain, unsweetened Greek yogurt to keep the phosphorus and potassium content low.
- Adjust the amount of honey to your taste preferences, or omit it entirely.
- You can also try other low-potassium fruit options, such as pears or berries, in place of the apples.

As always, it's important to consult with a registered dietitian or healthcare provider to ensure this recipe fits within your specific dietary needs for chronic kidney disease.

13. Low-potassium coleslaw

Ingredients:
- 2 cups shredded green cabbage
- 1 cup shredded red cabbage
- 2 tbsp low-fat or reduced-fat mayonnaise
- 1 tbsp white vinegar
- 1 tsp Dijon mustard
- 1 tsp honey (optional)
- 1/2 cup shredded carrots
- Salt and pepper to taste

Instructions:

1. In a large bowl, combine the shredded green cabbage, red cabbage, and carrots.

2. In a small bowl, whisk together the mayonnaise, white vinegar, Dijon mustard, and honey (if using).

3. Pour the dressing over the cabbage and carrot mixture and toss gently to coat.

4. Season with a small amount of salt and pepper to taste.

5. Chill the coleslaw in the refrigerator for at least 30 minutes before serving to allow the flavors to meld.

This recipe is a good option for seniors with chronic kidney disease for a few reasons:

- Cabbage and carrots are low-potassium vegetables, making them a good choice for kidney-friendly diets.

- The mayonnaise-based dressing is lower in phosphorus compared to creamy or dairy-based dressings.

- The vinegar and mustard add flavor without the need for high-sodium seasonings.
- Honey can provide a touch of sweetness without added sugars, if desired.

Some additional tips:

- Use a low-fat or reduced-fat mayonnaise to keep the calorie and saturated fat content lower.

- Adjust the amounts of the ingredients to suit your taste preferences.

- You can also try adding other low-potassium vegetables, such as radishes or jicama, to the coleslaw.

As always, it's important to consult with a registered dietitian or healthcare provider to ensure this recipe fits within your specific dietary needs for chronic kidney disease.

14. Carrot and raisin salad

Ingredients:
- 3 cups grated or shredded carrots
- 1/2 cup raisins
- 2 tbsp unsweetened almond milk
- 1 tbsp lemon juice
- 1 tsp honey (optional)
- Ground cinnamon (optional)

Instructions:
1. In a medium bowl, combine the grated or shredded carrots and raisins.

2. In a small bowl, whisk together the almond milk, lemon juice, and honey (if using).

3. Pour the dressing over the carrot and raisin mixture and toss gently to coat.

4. Sprinkle a small amount of ground cinnamon over the top, if desired.

5. Chill the salad in the refrigerator for at least 30 minutes before serving.

This recipe is a good option for seniors with chronic kidney disease for a few reasons:

- Carrots are a low-potassium vegetable, making them a good choice for kidney-friendly diets.

- Raisins are a low-potassium dried fruit option.

- Almond milk is lower in phosphorus and potassium compared to regular dairy milk.

- Lemon juice and cinnamon add flavor without the need for high-sodium seasonings.

Some additional tips:

- Adjust the amount of honey to your taste preferences, or omit it entirely.

- You can also try other low-potassium dried fruits, such as apricots or cranberries, in place of the raisins.

- The salad can be served as a side dish or a light snack.

As always, it's important to consult with a registered dietitian or healthcare provider to ensure this recipe fits within your specific dietary needs for chronic kidney disease.

15. Quinoa salad with cranberries and spinach

Ingredients:
- 1 cup cooked quinoa, cooled
- 1 cup fresh spinach, chopped
- 1/4 cup dried cranberries
- 2 tbsp unsweetened almond milk
- 1 tbsp lemon juice
- 1 tsp olive oil
- Salt and pepper to taste

Instructions:
1. In a medium bowl, combine the cooked quinoa, chopped spinach, and dried cranberries.

2. In a small bowl, whisk together the almond milk, lemon juice, and olive oil.

3. Pour the dressing over the quinoa mixture and toss gently to coat.

4. Season with a small amount of salt and pepper to taste.

5. Chill the salad in the refrigerator for at least 30 minutes before serving to allow the flavors to meld.

This recipe is a good option for seniors with chronic kidney disease for a few reasons:
- Quinoa is a whole grain that is low in phosphorus, making it a kidney-friendly choice.

- Spinach is a nutrient-dense green that is low in potassium.

- Dried cranberries are a low-potassium fruit option.

- Almond milk is lower in phosphorus and potassium compared to regular dairy milk.

- The lemon juice and olive oil provide a light, flavorful dressing without added sodium.

Some additional tips:
- Adjust the amounts of the ingredients to suit your taste preferences.

- You can also try other low-potassium vegetables, such as bell peppers or cucumber, in place of or in addition to the spinach. The salad can be served as a main dish or a side dish.

As always, it's important to consult with a registered dietitian or healthcare provider to ensure this recipe fits within your specific dietary needs for chronic kidney disease.

16. Spinach and strawberry salad

Ingredients:
- 4 cups fresh spinach leaves, washed and torn into bite-sized pieces
- 1 cup fresh strawberries, sliced
- 2 tbsp unsweetened almond milk
- 1 tbsp balsamic vinegar
- 1 tsp olive oil
- Salt and pepper to taste

Instructions:
1. In a large salad bowl, combine the spinach leaves and sliced strawberries.

2. In a small bowl, whisk together the almond milk, balsamic vinegar, and olive oil to make the dressing.

3. Pour the dressing over the spinach and strawberry mixture and toss gently to coat.

4. Season with a small amount of salt and pepper to taste. Serve the salad immediately.

This recipe is a good option for seniors with chronic kidney disease for a few reasons:

- Spinach is a nutrient-dense green that is low in potassium, making it a good choice for kidney-friendly diets.

- Strawberries are a low-potassium fruit option.

- Almond milk is lower in phosphorus and potassium compared to regular dairy milk.

- Balsamic vinegar and olive oil provide a light, flavorful dressing without added sodium.

Some additional tips:

- You can also try other low-potassium fruit options, such as blueberries or raspberries, in place of or in addition to the strawberries.

- Adjust the amounts of the ingredients to suit your taste preferences. The salad can be served as a main dish or a side dish.

As always, it's important to consult with a registered dietitian or healthcare provider to ensure this recipe fits within your specific dietary needs for chronic kidney disease.

17. Mixed greens with raspberries and almonds

Ingredients:
- 4 cups mixed greens (such as spinach, arugula, and kale)
- 1 cup fresh raspberries
- 2 tbsp sliced almonds
- 1 tbsp balsamic vinegar
- 1 tsp olive oil
- Salt and pepper to taste

Instructions:
1. In a large salad bowl, combine the mixed greens, fresh raspberries, and sliced almonds.

2. In a small bowl, whisk together the balsamic vinegar and olive oil to make the dressing.

3. Pour the dressing over the salad and toss gently to coat.

4. Season with a small amount of salt and pepper to taste.

5. Serve the salad immediately.

This recipe is a good option for seniors with chronic kidney disease for a few reasons:

- Mixed greens, such as spinach, arugula, and kale, are low in potassium and provide a nutrient-dense base for the salad.

- Raspberries are a low-potassium fruit option.

- Almonds provide a source of healthy fats without excessive phosphorus.

- Balsamic vinegar and olive oil create a light, flavorful dressing without added sodium.

Some additional tips:
- You can also try other low-potassium nuts or seeds, such as walnuts or pumpkin seeds, in place of or in addition to the almonds.

- Adjust the amounts of the ingredients to suit your taste preferences.

- The salad can be served as a main dish or a side dish.

As always, it's important to consult with a registered dietitian or healthcare provider to ensure this recipe fits within your specific dietary needs for chronic kidney disease.

18. Beet and arugula salad

Ingredients:
- 2 medium beets, peeled and sliced
- 4 cups fresh arugula
- 2 tbsp unsweetened almond milk
- 1 tbsp lemon juice
- 1 tsp olive oil
- Salt and pepper to taste

Instructions:
1. In a medium saucepan, bring water to a boil. Add the sliced beets and cook until tender, about 15-20 minutes. Drain and let cool.

2. In a large salad bowl, combine the cooked beet slices and fresh arugula.

3. In a small bowl, whisk together the almond milk, lemon juice, and olive oil to make the dressing.

4. Pour the dressing over the beet and arugula salad and toss gently to coat.

5. Season with a small amount of salt and pepper to taste. Serve the salad immediately.

This recipe is a good option for seniors with chronic kidney disease for a few reasons:

- Beets are a low-potassium vegetable, making them a good choice for kidney-friendly diets.

- Arugula is a nutrient-dense green that is also low in potassium.

- Almond milk is lower in phosphorus and potassium compared to regular dairy milk.

- Lemon juice and olive oil provide a light, flavorful dressing without added sodium.

Some additional tips:

- You can also try other low-potassium greens, such as spinach or kale, in place of or in addition to the arugula.
- Adjust the amounts of the ingredients to suit your taste preferences.
- The salad can be served as a main dish or a side dish.

As always, it's important to consult with a registered dietitian or healthcare provider to ensure this recipe fits within your specific dietary needs for chronic kidney disease.

19. Orzo pasta salad with fresh herbs

Ingredients:
- 1 cup uncooked orzo pasta
- 2 tbsp chopped fresh parsley
- 2 tbsp chopped fresh basil

- 2 tbsp unsweetened almond milk
- 1 tbsp lemon juice
- 1 tsp olive oil
- 1 tbsp chopped fresh dill
- Salt and pepper to taste

Instructions:

1. Cook the orzo pasta according to the package instructions. Drain and rinse with cold water to cool.

2. In a medium bowl, combine the cooked and cooled orzo pasta, chopped parsley, basil, and dill.

3. In a small bowl, whisk together the almond milk, lemon juice, and olive oil to make the dressing.

4. Pour the dressing over the orzo and herb mixture and toss gently to coat.

5. Season with a small amount of salt and pepper to taste.

6. Chill the pasta salad in the refrigerator for at least 30 minutes before serving to allow the flavors to meld.

This recipe is a good option for seniors with chronic kidney disease for a few reasons:

- Orzo is a type of small, rice-shaped pasta that is lower in phosphorus compared to other pasta varieties.
- Fresh herbs, such as parsley, basil, and dill, add flavor without the need for high-sodium seasonings.
- Almond milk is lower in phosphorus and potassium compared to regular dairy milk.
- Lemon juice and olive oil provide a light, flavorful dressing without added sodium.

Some additional tips:

- You can also try other low-potassium vegetables, such as diced cucumber or cherry tomatoes, in the salad.
- Adjust the amounts of the herbs and dressing to suit your taste preferences.
- The pasta salad can be served as a main dish or a side dish.

As always, it's important to consult with a registered dietitian or healthcare provider to ensure this recipe fits within your specific dietary needs for chronic kidney disease.

20. Cabbage and apple slaw

Ingredients:
- 2 cups shredded green cabbage
- 1 cup shredded red cabbage
- 1 medium apple, julienned or grated
- 2 tbsp unsweetened almond milk
- 1 tbsp apple cider vinegar
- 1 tsp Dijon mustard
- Salt and pepper to taste

Instructions:
1. In a large bowl, combine the shredded green cabbage, red cabbage, and julienned or grated apple.

2. In a small bowl, whisk together the almond milk, apple cider vinegar, and Dijon mustard to make the dressing.

3. Pour the dressing over the cabbage and apple mixture and toss gently to coat.

4. Season with a small amount of salt and pepper to taste.

5. Chill the slaw in the refrigerator for at least 30 minutes before serving to allow the flavors to meld.

This recipe is a good option for seniors with chronic kidney disease for a few reasons:

- Cabbage is a low-potassium vegetable, making it a good choice for kidney-friendly diets.
- Apples are a low-potassium fruit option.
- Almond milk is lower in phosphorus and potassium compared to regular dairy milk.
- Apple cider vinegar and Dijon mustard add flavor without the need for high-sodium seasonings.

Some additional tips:

- You can also try other low-potassium vegetables, such as carrots or radishes, in the slaw.
- Adjust the amounts of the ingredients to suit your taste preferences.
- The slaw can be served as a side dish or a topping for grilled or roasted meats.

As always, it's important to consult with a registered dietitian or healthcare provider to ensure this recipe fits within your specific dietary needs for chronic kidney disease.

21. Low-sodium chicken noodle soup

Ingredients:
- 4 cups low-sodium chicken broth
- 1 boneless, skinless chicken breast, cooked and shredded
- 1 cup cooked whole wheat egg noodles
- 1 cup diced carrots
- 1 cup diced celery
- 1 tbsp chopped fresh parsley
- 1 tsp dried thyme
- Salt and pepper to taste

Instructions:
1. In a large saucepan, bring the low-sodium chicken broth to a simmer over medium heat.

2. Add the shredded chicken, cooked noodles, diced carrots, and diced celery to the broth. Simmer for 10-15 minutes, or until the vegetables are tender.

3. Stir in the chopped fresh parsley and dried thyme.

4. Season with a small amount of salt and pepper to taste. Serve the soup hot.

This recipe is a good option for seniors with chronic kidney disease for a few reasons:

- Low-sodium chicken broth is lower in sodium compared to regular broth or stock.
- Chicken is a lean protein source that is low in phosphorus.
- Whole wheat egg noodles are a good source of complex carbohydrates without excessive phosphorus.
- Carrots and celery are low-potassium vegetables that add flavor and nutrition.
- Fresh parsley and dried thyme provide seasoning without the need for high-sodium additives.

Some additional tips:

- You can also try other low-potassium vegetables, such as spinach or zucchini, in the soup.
- Adjust the amounts of the ingredients to suit your taste preferences.
- The soup can be a comforting and nourishing meal on its own or served with a side salad.

As always, it's important to consult with a registered dietitian or healthcare provider to ensure this recipe fits within your specific dietary needs for chronic kidney disease.

22. Vegetable barley soup

Ingredients:
- 4 cups low-sodium vegetable broth
- 1/2 cup uncooked pearl barley
- 1 cup diced carrots
- 1 cup diced celery
- 1 cup diced zucchini
- 1 cup diced tomatoes (no-salt-added)
- 2 tbsp chopped fresh parsley
- 1 tsp dried thyme
- Salt and pepper to taste

Instructions:
1. In a large saucepan, bring the low-sodium vegetable broth to a boil over medium-high heat.

2. Add the uncooked pearl barley, diced carrots, celery, and zucchini to the broth. Reduce heat to medium-low and simmer for 20-25 minutes, or until the barley and vegetables are tender.

3. Stir in the diced no-salt-added tomatoes, chopped fresh parsley, and dried thyme.

4. Season with a small amount of salt and pepper to taste. Serve the soup hot.

This recipe is a good option for seniors with chronic kidney disease for a few reasons:

- Low-sodium vegetable broth is lower in sodium compared to regular broth or stock.
- Pearl barley is a whole grain that is low in phosphorus.
- Carrots, celery, zucchini, and tomatoes are all low-potassium vegetables that add flavor and nutrition to the soup.
- Fresh parsley and dried thyme provide seasoning without the need for high-sodium additives.

Some additional tips:
- You can also try other low-potassium vegetables, such as spinach or green beans, in the soup.
- Adjust the amounts of the ingredients to suit your taste preferences.
- The soup can be a comforting and nourishing meal on its own or served with a side salad.

As always, it's important to consult with a registered dietitian or healthcare provider to ensure this recipe fits within your specific dietary needs for chronic kidney disease.

23. Creamy cauliflower soup

Ingredients:
- 1 head of cauliflower, cut into florets
- 2 cups unsweetened almond milk
- 1 tbsp olive oil
- 1 onion, diced
- 2 cloves garlic, minced
- 1 tsp dried thyme
- Salt and pepper to taste

Instructions:
1. In a large saucepan, bring 2 cups of water to a boil. Add the cauliflower florets and cook for 10-15 minutes, until very tender.

2. Drain the cauliflower and transfer it to a blender. Add the almond milk and blend until smooth and creamy.

3. In the same saucepan, heat the olive oil over medium heat. Add the diced onion and minced garlic. Cook for 5-7 minutes, until the onion is translucent.

4. Pour the blended cauliflower mixture into the saucepan with the onions and garlic. Stir in the dried thyme.

5. Simmer the soup for 5-10 minutes, stirring occasionally, until heated through. Season with a small amount of salt and pepper to taste. Serve the soup hot.

This recipe is a good option for seniors with chronic kidney disease for a few reasons:

- Cauliflower is a low-potassium vegetable that is also low in phosphorus.
- Unsweetened almond milk is lower in phosphorus and potassium compared to regular dairy milk.
- The soup is creamy and comforting without the need for high-sodium ingredients or dairy products.
- Dried thyme adds flavor without the need for high-sodium seasonings.

Some additional tips:

- You can also try adding other low-potassium vegetables, such as spinach or zucchini, to the soup.
- Adjust the amounts of the ingredients to suit your taste preferences.
- The soup can be a satisfying and nourishing meal on its own or served with a side salad.

24. Carrot and ginger soup

Ingredients:
- 1 lb carrots, peeled and sliced
- 1 onion, diced
- 2 cloves garlic, minced
- 1 tbsp grated fresh ginger
- 4 cups low-sodium vegetable broth
- 1 cup unsweetened almond milk
- 1 tsp ground coriander
- Salt and pepper to taste

Instructions:
1. In a large saucepan, sauté the diced onion and minced garlic in a small amount of olive oil over medium heat for 3-4 minutes, until translucent.

2. Add the sliced carrots, grated ginger, and ground coriander. Sauté for an additional 2-3 minutes.

3. Pour in the low-sodium vegetable broth and bring the mixture to a boil. Reduce heat and simmer for 20-25 minutes, or until the carrots are very tender.

4. Remove the soup from heat and use an immersion blender (or transfer to a regular blender) to puree the soup until smooth and creamy.

5. Stir in the unsweetened almond milk and season with a small amount of salt and pepper to taste. Serve the soup hot.

This recipe is a good option for seniors with chronic kidney disease for a few reasons:

- Carrots are a low-potassium vegetable that are also low in phosphorus.
- Ginger adds flavor without the need for high-sodium seasonings.
- Unsweetened almond milk is lower in phosphorus and potassium compared to regular dairy milk.
- The soup is creamy and comforting without the use of high-sodium ingredients or dairy products.

Some additional tips:
- You can also try adding other low-potassium vegetables, such as celery or zucchini, to the soup.
- Adjust the amounts of the ingredients to suit your taste preferences.
- The soup can be a satisfying and nourishing meal on its own or served with a side salad.

25. Butternut squash soup

Ingredients:
- 1 medium butternut squash, peeled, seeded, and cubed
- 1 onion, diced
- 2 cloves garlic, minced
- 4 cups low-sodium vegetable broth
- 1 cup unsweetened almond milk
- 1 tsp ground cinnamon
- 1/2 tsp ground nutmeg
- Salt and pepper to taste

Instructions:
1. In a large saucepan or Dutch oven, sauté the diced onion and minced garlic in a small amount of olive oil over medium heat for 3-4 minutes, until translucent.

2. Add the cubed butternut squash and low-sodium vegetable broth to the pan. Bring the mixture to a boil, then reduce heat and simmer for 20-25 minutes, or until the squash is very tender.

3. Remove the pan from heat and use an immersion blender (or transfer to a regular blender) to puree the soup until smooth and creamy.

4. Stir in the unsweetened almond milk, ground cinnamon, and ground nutmeg.

5. Season with a small amount of salt and pepper to taste. Serve the soup hot.

This recipe is a good option for seniors with chronic kidney disease for a few reasons:

- Butternut squash is a low-potassium vegetable that is also low in phosphorus.
- Unsweetened almond milk is lower in phosphorus and potassium compared to regular dairy milk.
- Cinnamon and nutmeg add warmth and flavor without the need for high-sodium seasonings.
- The soup is creamy and comforting without the use of high-sodium ingredients or dairy products.

Some additional tips:
- You can also try adding other low-potassium vegetables, such as carrots or celery, to the soup.
- Adjust the amounts of the spices to suit your taste preferences.
- The soup can be a satisfying and nourishing meal on its own or served with a side salad.

26. Low-sodium beef stew

Ingredients:
- 1 lb lean beef stew meat, cubed
- 2 cups low-sodium beef broth
- 2 cups diced potatoes
- 1 cup diced carrots
- 1 cup diced celery
- 1 onion, diced
- 2 cloves garlic, minced
- 1 tsp dried thyme
- 1 bay leaf
- Salt and pepper to taste

Instructions:
1. In a large pot or Dutch oven, brown the cubed beef over medium-high heat. Drain any excess fat.

2. Add the low-sodium beef broth, diced potatoes, carrots, celery, onion, and garlic to the pot. Stir in the dried thyme and bay leaf.

3. Bring the mixture to a boil, then reduce heat and simmer for 45-60 minutes, or until the beef and vegetables are tender.

4. Remove the bay leaf. Season the stew with a small amount of salt and pepper to taste. Serve the stew hot.

This recipe is a good option for seniors with chronic kidney disease for a few reasons:

- Lean beef is a good source of protein without excessive phosphorus.
- Low-sodium beef broth helps to keep the sodium content lower compared to regular broth.
- Potatoes, carrots, and celery are all low-potassium vegetables that add nutrition and flavor to the stew.
- Dried thyme provides seasoning without the need for high-sodium additives.

Some additional tips:

- You can also try adding other low-potassium vegetables, such as green beans or zucchini, to the stew.
- Adjust the amounts of the ingredients to suit your taste preferences.
- The stew can be a comforting and nourishing meal on its own or served with a side salad.

27. Cabbage soup

Ingredients:
- 1 head of green cabbage, chopped
- 1 onion, diced
- 2 carrots, diced
- 2 celery stalks, diced
- 4 cups low-sodium vegetable broth
- 1 (15 oz) can no-salt-added diced tomatoes
- 2 tbsp chopped fresh parsley
- 1 tsp dried thyme
- Salt and pepper to taste

Instructions:
1. In a large pot or Dutch oven, sauté the diced onion over medium heat until translucent, about 3-4 minutes.

2. Add the chopped cabbage, diced carrots, and diced celery to the pot. Sauté for an additional 5 minutes.

3. Pour in the low-sodium vegetable broth and the can of no-salt-added diced tomatoes. Bring the mixture to a boil.

4. Reduce heat and let the soup simmer for 20-25 minutes, or until the vegetables are tender.

5. Stir in the chopped fresh parsley and dried thyme. Season the soup with a small amount of salt and pepper to taste. Serve the cabbage soup hot.

This recipe is a good option for seniors with chronic kidney disease for a few reasons:
- Cabbage, carrots, and celery are all low-potassium vegetables that are also low in phosphorus.
- Low-sodium vegetable broth helps to keep the sodium content lower compared to regular broth.
- No-salt-added diced tomatoes provide flavor without excessive sodium.
- Fresh parsley and dried thyme add seasoning without the need for high-sodium additives.

Some additional tips:
- You can also try adding other low-potassium vegetables, such as zucchini or spinach, to the soup.
- Adjust the amounts of the ingredients to suit your taste preferences.
- The soup can be a comforting and nourishing meal on its own or served with a side salad.

28. Pumpkin soup

Ingredients:
- 1 (15 oz) can pumpkin puree
- 4 cups low-sodium vegetable broth
- 1 cup unsweetened almond milk
- 1 onion, diced
- 2 cloves garlic, minced
- 1 tsp ground cinnamon
- 1/2 tsp ground ginger
- Salt and pepper to taste

Instructions:

1. In a large saucepan, sauté the diced onion and minced garlic in a small amount of olive oil over medium heat for 3-4 minutes, until translucent.

2. Add the canned pumpkin puree, low-sodium vegetable broth, and unsweetened almond milk to the saucepan. Stir to combine.

3. Stir in the ground cinnamon and ground ginger.

4. Bring the soup to a simmer and let it cook for 10-15 minutes, stirring occasionally, until heated through.

5. Use an immersion blender (or transfer to a regular blender) to puree the soup until smooth and creamy.

6. Season the soup with a small amount of salt and pepper to taste. Serve the pumpkin soup hot.

This recipe is a good option for seniors with chronic kidney disease for a few reasons:

- Pumpkin is a low-potassium vegetable that is also low in phosphorus.
- Unsweetened almond milk is lower in phosphorus and potassium compared to regular dairy milk.
- Cinnamon and ginger add warmth and flavor without the need for high-sodium seasonings.
- The soup is creamy and comforting without the use of high-sodium ingredients or dairy products.

Some additional tips:

- You can also try adding other low-potassium vegetables, such as carrots or celery, to the soup.
- Adjust the amounts of the spices to suit your taste preferences.
- The soup can be a satisfying and nourishing meal on its own or served with a side salad.

29. Broccoli and rice soup

Ingredients:
- 1 cup uncooked brown rice
- 4 cups low-sodium vegetable broth
- 1 head of broccoli, chopped into florets
- 1 onion, diced
- 2 cloves garlic, minced
- 1 cup unsweetened almond milk
- 1 tsp dried thyme
- Salt and pepper to taste

Instructions:
1. In a medium saucepan, cook the brown rice according to package instructions. Drain and set aside.

2. In a large pot or Dutch oven, sauté the diced onion and minced garlic in a small amount of olive oil over medium heat for 3-4 minutes, until translucent.

3. Add the chopped broccoli florets and low-sodium vegetable broth to the pot. Bring the mixture to a boil, then reduce heat and simmer for 10-15 minutes, until the broccoli is tender.

4. Stir in the cooked brown rice and unsweetened almond milk. Heat through.

5. Stir in the dried thyme and season with a small amount of salt and pepper to taste. Serve the broccoli and rice soup hot.

This recipe is a good option for seniors with chronic kidney disease for a few reasons:

- Broccoli is a low-potassium vegetable that is also low in phosphorus.
- Brown rice is a whole grain that is lower in phosphorus compared to white rice.
- Unsweetened almond milk is lower in phosphorus and potassium compared to regular dairy milk.
- Dried thyme adds flavor without the need for high-sodium seasonings.

Some additional tips:

- You can also try adding other low-potassium vegetables, such as spinach or zucchini, to the soup.
- Adjust the amounts of the ingredients to suit your taste preferences.
- The soup can be a comforting and nourishing meal on its own or served with a side salad.

30. Leek and potato soup

Ingredients:
- 2 leeks, sliced (white and light green parts only)
- 2 medium potatoes, peeled and diced
- 4 cups low-sodium chicken or vegetable broth
- 1 cup unsweetened almond milk or low-fat milk
- 2 tbsp fresh parsley, chopped
- Salt and pepper to taste

Instructions:
1. In a large pot, sauté the sliced leeks in a small amount of oil or butter over medium heat until softened, about 5 minutes.

2. Add the diced potatoes and broth. Bring to a boil, then reduce heat and simmer for 15-20 minutes, until potatoes are tender.

3. Use an immersion blender or regular blender to puree the soup until smooth.

4. Stir in the almond or low-fat milk and parsley. Season with salt and pepper to taste.

5. Serve warm.

Tips:
- Use low-sodium broth to keep sodium content down.

- Avoid adding high-potassium ingredients like spinach or mushrooms.

- Adjust portion sizes as needed to fit individual dietary needs.

- This soup is easy to digest and provides nutrients like vitamin C, vitamin K, and fiber.

31. Grilled chicken with lemon and herbs

Ingredients:
- 4 boneless, skinless chicken breasts
- 2 tbsp olive oil
- 2 tbsp fresh lemon juice
- 1 tsp dried oregano
- 1 tsp dried basil
- 1/2 tsp garlic powder
- Salt and pepper to taste

Instructions:
1. In a shallow dish, combine the olive oil, lemon juice, oregano, basil, and garlic powder. Add the chicken breasts and turn to coat both sides.

2. Cover and marinate in the refrigerator for 30 minutes to 1 hour.

3. Preheat grill or grill pan to medium-high heat.

4. Grill the chicken for 5-7 minutes per side, or until cooked through and no longer pink in the center.

5. Transfer the grilled chicken to a plate and season with salt and pepper to taste. Serve immediately.

Tips:
- Use low-sodium seasonings or omit salt if needed to reduce sodium intake.

- Pair the chicken with low-potassium side dishes like steamed broccoli, roasted cauliflower, or a small portion of brown rice.

- Avoid high-potassium marinades or sauces.

- Adjust cooking time as needed to ensure the chicken is cooked through.

This recipe provides a flavorful, protein-rich meal that is suitable for seniors with chronic kidney disease. The lemon and herbs add flavor without the need for high-sodium ingredients.

32. Baked cod with dill and lemon

Ingredients:
- 4 cod fillets (about 4-6 oz each)
- 2 tbsp olive oil
- 2 tbsp fresh lemon juice
- 1 tsp dried dill
- 1/4 tsp garlic powder
- Salt and pepper to taste

Instructions:
1. Preheat the oven to 400°F.

2. Place the cod fillets in a baking dish or on a parchment-lined baking sheet.

3. In a small bowl, whisk together the olive oil, lemon juice, dried dill, and garlic powder.

4. Drizzle the lemon-dill mixture over the cod fillets, making sure to coat them evenly.

5. Season the cod with salt and pepper to taste.

6. Bake for 12-15 minutes, or until the cod is opaque and flakes easily with a fork.

7. Serve the baked cod immediately, garnished with additional fresh dill if desired.

Tips:
- Use low-sodium or no-salt-added seasonings to keep sodium content low.

- Pair the baked cod with steamed vegetables, such as broccoli or asparagus, and a small portion of a low-potassium starch, like white rice or quinoa.

- Avoid high-potassium sauces or toppings, such as butter or hollandaise.

- Adjust cooking time as needed to ensure the cod is cooked through but not overcooked.

This recipe provides a simple, flavorful way to prepare cod that is suitable for seniors with chronic kidney disease. The lemon and dill add freshness without the need for high-sodium ingredients.

33. Turkey meatballs with rice

Ingredients:
- 1 lb ground turkey
- 1/4 cup cooked white rice
- 1 egg, lightly beaten
- 2 tbsp fresh parsley, chopped
- 1 tsp garlic powder
- 1/2 tsp onion powder
- Salt and pepper to taste
- 2 cups cooked white rice, for serving

Instructions:
1. Preheat the oven to 400°F.

2. In a large bowl, combine the ground turkey, cooked rice, egg, parsley, garlic powder, and onion powder. Season with salt and pepper to taste.

3. Using your hands, gently form the mixture into 1-inch meatballs, being careful not to overmix.

4. Place the meatballs on a parchment-lined baking sheet.

5. Bake for 18-20 minutes, or until the meatballs are cooked through and no longer pink in the center. Serve the turkey meatballs over the cooked white rice.

Tips:

- Use low-sodium or no-salt-added seasonings to keep sodium content low.

- Avoid adding high-potassium ingredients like tomato sauce or cheese.

- Adjust portion sizes as needed to fit individual dietary needs.

- This dish provides a good source of protein from the turkey and a moderate amount of carbohydrates from the rice.

This recipe for turkey meatballs with rice is a simple, protein-rich meal that can be suitable for seniors with chronic kidney disease. The use of white rice and low-sodium seasonings helps to keep the dish within recommended dietary guidelines.

34. Herb-crusted tilapia

Ingredients:
- 4 tilapia fillets (about 4-6 oz each)
- 2 tbsp panko breadcrumbs
- 1 tbsp grated Parmesan cheese (optional)
- 1 tsp dried parsley
- 1 tsp dried basil
- 1/2 tsp garlic powder
- 1/4 tsp paprika
- 2 tbsp olive oil
- Salt and pepper to taste

Instructions:
1. Preheat the oven to 400°F.

2. In a shallow bowl, mix together the panko breadcrumbs, Parmesan cheese (if using), parsley, basil, garlic powder, and paprika.

3. Brush the tilapia fillets with the olive oil and season with salt and pepper.

4. Dip the tilapia fillets into the breadcrumb mixture, pressing gently to help the coating adhere.

5. Place the coated tilapia fillets on a parchment-lined baking sheet.

6. Bake for 12-15 minutes, or until the fish is opaque and flakes easily with a fork.

7. Serve the herb-crusted tilapia immediately.

Tips:
- Use low-sodium or no-salt-added seasonings to keep sodium content low.
- Omit the Parmesan cheese if you need to further reduce sodium.
- Pair the tilapia with steamed vegetables, such as broccoli or asparagus, and a small portion of a low-potassium starch, like white rice or quinoa.
- Adjust cooking time as needed to ensure the tilapia is cooked through but not overcooked.

This recipe for herb-crusted tilapia provides a flavorful, baked fish dish that is suitable for seniors with chronic kidney disease. The use of low-sodium seasonings and the avoidance of high-potassium ingredients make it a kidney-friendly option.

35. Grilled shrimp with garlic and parsley

Ingredients:
- 1 lb large shrimp, peeled and deveined
- 2 tbsp olive oil
- 3 cloves garlic, minced
- 2 tbsp fresh parsley, chopped
- 1 tbsp lemon juice
- Salt and pepper to taste

Instructions:
1. In a large bowl, combine the shrimp, olive oil, garlic, parsley, and lemon juice. Toss to coat the shrimp evenly.

2. Season the shrimp with salt and pepper to taste.

3. Preheat a grill or grill pan to medium-high heat.

4. Thread the shrimp onto skewers, leaving a little space between each shrimp.

5. Grill the shrimp for 2-3 minutes per side, or until they are opaque and cooked through.

6. Serve the grilled shrimp immediately, garnished with additional parsley if desired.

Tips:
- Use low-sodium or no-salt-added seasonings to keep sodium content low.

- Avoid high-potassium marinades or sauces.

- Pair the grilled shrimp with a side of steamed vegetables, such as broccoli or asparagus, and a small portion of a low-potassium starch, like white rice or quinoa.

- Adjust cooking time as needed to ensure the shrimp are cooked through but not overcooked.

This recipe for grilled shrimp with garlic and parsley provides a flavorful, protein-rich dish that is suitable for seniors with chronic kidney disease. The use of simple seasonings and the avoidance of high-sodium or high-potassium ingredients make it a kidney-friendly option.

36. Baked chicken thighs with rosemary

Ingredients:
- 6 bone-in, skin-on chicken thighs
- 2 tbsp olive oil
- 2 tsp dried rosemary
- 1 tsp garlic powder
- 1/2 tsp onion powder
- Salt and pepper to taste

Instructions:
1. Preheat the oven to 400°F.

2. Pat the chicken thighs dry with paper towels and place them in a baking dish or on a parchment-lined baking sheet.

3. In a small bowl, mix together the olive oil, dried rosemary, garlic powder, and onion powder.

4. Brush the rosemary-garlic mixture over the chicken thighs, making sure to coat them evenly.

5. Season the chicken with salt and pepper to taste.

6. Bake the chicken thighs for 35-40 minutes, or until the internal temperature reaches 165°F and the skin is crispy. Serve the baked chicken thighs immediately.

Tips:
- Use low-sodium or no-salt-added seasonings to keep sodium content low.

- Avoid high-potassium ingredients like lemon or herbs like parsley.

- Pair the baked chicken with steamed vegetables, such as green beans or carrots, and a small portion of a low-potassium starch, like white rice or quinoa.

- Adjust cooking time as needed to ensure the chicken is cooked through but not overcooked.

This recipe for baked chicken thighs with rosemary provides a flavorful, protein-rich dish that is suitable for seniors with chronic kidney disease. The use of simple, low-sodium seasonings and the avoidance of high-potassium ingredients make it a kidney-friendly option.

37. Low-sodium beef stir-fry with vegetables

Ingredients:
- 1 lb beef sirloin, thinly sliced
- 2 tbsp low-sodium soy sauce or tamari
- 1 tbsp rice vinegar
- 1 tsp sesame oil
- 1 tsp cornstarch
- 2 tbsp olive oil
- 2 cloves garlic, minced
- 1 inch fresh ginger, peeled and grated
- 1 cup broccoli florets
- 1 cup sliced mushrooms
- 1 cup sliced bell peppers
- 1/2 cup sliced water chestnuts
- 2 cups cooked brown rice, for serving

Instructions:
1. In a bowl, combine the sliced beef, low-sodium soy sauce, rice vinegar, sesame oil, and cornstarch. Toss to coat the beef and set aside.

2. Heat the olive oil in a large skillet or wok over high heat.

3. Add the garlic and ginger and stir-fry for 30 seconds until fragrant.

4. Add the marinated beef and stir-fry for 2-3 minutes, until the beef is no longer pink.

5. Add the broccoli, mushrooms, bell peppers, and water chestnuts. Stir-fry for an additional 3-4 minutes, until the vegetables are tender-crisp.

6. Serve the beef and vegetable stir-fry over the cooked brown rice.

Tips:
- Use low-sodium soy sauce or tamari to keep sodium content low.

- Avoid high-potassium vegetables like spinach or tomatoes.

- Adjust portion sizes as needed to fit individual dietary needs.

- This dish provides a good source of protein, fiber, and various vitamins and minerals.

This low-sodium beef stir-fry with vegetables is a flavorful and nutritious meal that can be suitable for seniors with chronic kidney disease. The use of low-sodium soy sauce and the avoidance of high-potassium ingredients make it a kidney-friendly option.

38. Herb-roasted pork tenderloin

Ingredients:
- 1 lb pork tenderloin
- 2 tbsp olive oil
- 1 tsp dried thyme
- 1 tsp dried rosemary
- 1 tsp garlic powder
- 1/2 tsp onion powder
- Salt and pepper to taste

Instructions:
1. Preheat the oven to 400°F.

2. Pat the pork tenderloin dry with paper towels and place it in a baking dish or on a parchment-lined baking sheet.

3. In a small bowl, mix together the olive oil, dried thyme, dried rosemary, garlic powder, and onion powder.

4. Rub the herb-oil mixture all over the pork tenderloin, making sure to coat it evenly.

5. Season the pork with salt and pepper to taste.

6. Roast the pork tenderloin for 25-30 minutes, or until the internal temperature reaches 145°F. Let the pork rest for 5-10 minutes before slicing and serving.

Tips:

- Use low-sodium or no-salt-added seasonings to keep sodium content low.

- Avoid high-potassium herbs like parsley or cilantro.

- Pair the roasted pork with steamed vegetables, such as green beans or carrots, and a small

portion of a low-potassium starch, like white rice or quinoa.

- Adjust cooking time as needed to ensure the pork is cooked through but not overcooked.

This recipe for herb-roasted pork tenderloin provides a flavorful, protein-rich dish that is suitable for seniors with chronic kidney disease. The use of simple, low-sodium seasonings and the avoidance of high-potassium ingredients make it a kidney-friendly option.

39. Spaghetti squash with tomato sauce

Ingredients:
- 1 medium spaghetti squash, halved lengthwise and seeded
- 1 tbsp olive oil
- 1 can (14.5 oz) no-salt-added diced tomatoes
- 2 cloves garlic, minced
- 1 tsp dried basil
- 1/4 tsp dried oregano
- Salt and pepper to taste

Instructions:
1. Preheat the oven to 400°F.

2. Place the spaghetti squash halves cut-side down on a baking sheet. Bake for 40-50 minutes, or until the squash is tender and easily shreds with a fork.

3. In a medium saucepan, heat the olive oil over medium heat. Add the garlic and sauté for 1 minute, until fragrant.

4. Add the no-salt-added diced tomatoes, dried basil, and dried oregano. Simmer the sauce for 10-15 minutes, stirring occasionally, until slightly thickened.

5. Season the tomato sauce with salt and pepper to taste. Use a fork to shred the spaghetti squash flesh into strands. Serve the spaghetti squash strands topped with the tomato sauce.

Tips:
- Use no-salt-added or low-sodium canned tomatoes to keep sodium content low.

- Avoid high-potassium ingredients like fresh herbs or cheese.

- Adjust portion sizes as needed to fit individual dietary needs.

- This dish provides a good source of fiber, vitamins, and minerals.

This recipe for spaghetti squash with tomato sauce is a kidney-friendly, low-carbohydrate alternative to traditional pasta dishes. The use of no-salt-added tomatoes and the avoidance of high-potassium ingredients make it a suitable option for seniors with chronic kidney disease.

40. Lemon pepper salmon

Ingredients:
- 4 salmon fillets (about 4-6 oz each)
- 2 tbsp olive oil
- 2 tbsp lemon juice
- 1 tsp lemon zest
- 1 tsp ground black pepper
- 1/4 tsp salt (optional)

Instructions:
1. Preheat the oven to 400°F.

2. Place the salmon fillets in a baking dish or on a parchment-lined baking sheet.

3. In a small bowl, whisk together the olive oil, lemon juice, lemon zest, and black pepper.

4. Drizzle the lemon-pepper mixture over the salmon fillets, making sure to coat them evenly.

5. If desired, sprinkle a small amount of salt over the salmon (use sparingly to keep sodium low).

6. Bake the salmon for 12-15 minutes, or until it flakes easily with a fork and is cooked through. Serve the lemon pepper salmon immediately.

Tips:
- Use low-sodium or no-salt-added seasonings to keep sodium content low.

- Avoid high-potassium herbs or sauces.

- Pair the salmon with steamed vegetables, such as broccoli or asparagus, and a small portion of a low-potassium starch, like white rice or quinoa.

- Adjust cooking time as needed to ensure the salmon is cooked through but not overcooked.

This recipe for lemon pepper salmon provides a flavorful, protein-rich dish that is suitable for seniors with chronic kidney disease. The use of lemon and black pepper adds flavor without the need for high-sodium ingredients, making it a kidney-friendly option.

41. Steamed green beans with almonds

Ingredients:
- 1 lb fresh green beans, trimmed
- 1 tbsp olive oil
- 2 tbsp sliced almonds
- 1 tsp lemon zest
- Salt and pepper to taste

Instructions:
1. Fill a large pot with 1-2 inches of water and bring it to a boil.

2. Place the trimmed green beans in a steamer basket and lower it into the pot. Cover and steam the green beans for 5-7 minutes, or until they are tender-crisp.

3. Drain the steamed green beans and transfer them to a serving bowl.

4. In a small skillet, heat the olive oil over medium heat. Add the sliced almonds and sauté for 2-3 minutes, stirring frequently, until the almonds are lightly toasted.

5. Remove the skillet from the heat and stir in the lemon zest.

6. Pour the toasted almond mixture over the steamed green beans and toss to combine.

7. Season the green beans with salt and pepper to taste.

8. Serve the steamed green beans with almonds immediately.

Tips:
- Use low-sodium or no-salt-added seasonings to keep sodium content low.

- Avoid high-potassium ingredients like garlic or onions.

- Adjust portion sizes as needed to fit individual dietary needs.

- This dish provides a good source of fiber, vitamins, and healthy fats from the almonds.

This recipe for steamed green beans with almonds is a simple, flavorful side dish that is suitable for seniors with chronic kidney disease. The use of lemon zest and toasted almonds adds flavor without the need for high-sodium or high-potassium ingredients.

42. Roasted Brussels sprouts

Ingredients:
- 1 lb Brussels sprouts, trimmed and halved
- 2 tbsp olive oil
- 1 tsp dried thyme
- 1/2 tsp garlic powder
- Salt and pepper to taste

Instructions:
1. Preheat the oven to 400°F.

2. In a large bowl, toss the trimmed and halved Brussels sprouts with the olive oil, dried thyme, and garlic powder.

3. Spread the Brussels sprouts in a single layer on a parchment-lined baking sheet.

4. Roast the Brussels sprouts for 20-25 minutes, tossing halfway, until they are tender and lightly browned.

5. Season the roasted Brussels sprouts with salt and pepper to taste. Serve the roasted Brussels sprouts immediately.

Tips:
- Use low-sodium or no-salt-added seasonings to keep sodium content low.

- Avoid high-potassium ingredients like lemon juice or Parmesan cheese.

- Adjust portion sizes as needed to fit individual dietary needs.

- This dish provides a good source of fiber, vitamins, and minerals.

This recipe for roasted Brussels sprouts is a simple, flavorful side dish that is suitable for seniors with chronic kidney disease. The use of basic seasonings like thyme and garlic powder adds flavor without the need for high-sodium or high-potassium ingredients.

43. Baked zucchini with garlic

Ingredients:
- 2 medium zucchini, sliced into 1/2-inch rounds
- 2 tbsp olive oil
- 2 cloves garlic, minced
- 1 tsp dried oregano
- Salt and pepper to taste

Instructions:
1. Preheat the oven to 400°F.

2. In a large bowl, toss the zucchini slices with the olive oil, minced garlic, and dried oregano. Season with salt and pepper to taste.

3. Spread the seasoned zucchini slices in a single layer on a parchment-lined baking sheet.

4. Bake the zucchini for 15-20 minutes, flipping halfway, until tender and lightly browned.

5. Serve the baked zucchini with garlic immediately.

Tips:
- Use low-sodium or no-salt-added seasonings to keep sodium content low.

- Avoid high-potassium ingredients like cheese or fresh herbs.

- Adjust portion sizes as needed to fit individual dietary needs.

- This dish provides a good source of vitamins, minerals, and fiber.

This recipe for baked zucchini with garlic is a simple, flavorful side dish that is suitable for seniors with chronic kidney disease. The use of garlic and dried oregano adds flavor without the need for high-sodium or high-potassium ingredients.

44. Mashed cauliflower

Ingredients:
- 1 head of cauliflower, cut into florets
- 2 tbsp unsweetened almond milk or low-fat milk
- 1 tbsp olive oil
- 1 tsp garlic powder
- 1/4 tsp onion powder
- Salt and pepper to taste

Instructions:
1. In a large pot, bring 1-2 inches of water to a boil. Add the cauliflower florets, cover, and steam for 10-15 minutes, or until the cauliflower is very tender.

2. Drain the steamed cauliflower and transfer it to a food processor or high-powered blender.

3. Add the almond milk (or low-fat milk), olive oil, garlic powder, and onion powder. Blend or process the mixture until it is smooth and creamy.

4. Season the mashed cauliflower with salt and pepper to taste. Serve the mashed cauliflower warm.

Tips:

- Use low-sodium or no-salt-added seasonings to keep sodium content low.

- Avoid high-potassium ingredients like butter or cheese.

- Adjust portion sizes as needed to fit individual dietary needs.

- This dish provides a good source of vitamins, minerals, and fiber.

This recipe for mashed cauliflower is a low-carbohydrate, kidney-friendly alternative to traditional mashed potatoes. The use of almond milk or low-fat milk, along with simple seasonings, makes it a suitable option for seniors with chronic kidney disease.

45. Steamed asparagus with lemon

Ingredients:
- 1 lb fresh asparagus, trimmed
- 1 tbsp olive oil
- 1 tbsp lemon juice
- 1/2 tsp lemon zest
- Salt and pepper to taste

Instructions:

1. Fill a large pot with 1-2 inches of water and bring it to a boil.

2. Place the trimmed asparagus in a steamer basket and lower it into the pot. Cover and steam the asparagus for 5-7 minutes, or until they are tender-crisp.

3. Drain the steamed asparagus and transfer them to a serving dish.

4. In a small bowl, whisk together the olive oil, lemon juice, and lemon zest.

5. Drizzle the lemon-olive oil mixture over the steamed asparagus and toss to coat.

6. Season the asparagus with salt and pepper to taste.

7. Serve the steamed asparagus with lemon immediately.

Tips:

- Use low-sodium or no-salt-added seasonings to keep sodium content low.

- Avoid high-potassium ingredients like garlic or onions.

- Adjust portion sizes as needed to fit individual dietary needs.

- This dish provides a good source of vitamins, minerals, and fiber.

This recipe for steamed asparagus with lemon is a simple, flavorful side dish that is suitable for seniors with chronic kidney disease. The use of lemon juice and zest adds flavor without the need for high-sodium or high-potassium ingredients.

46. Roasted bell peppers

Ingredients:
- 4 bell peppers (mix of red, yellow, and/or orange)
- 2 tbsp olive oil
- 1 tsp dried oregano
- 1/4 tsp garlic powder
- Salt and pepper to taste

Instructions:
1. Preheat the oven to 400°F.

2. Cut the bell peppers in half lengthwise and remove the seeds and membranes.

3. Arrange the bell pepper halves, cut-side up, on a parchment-lined baking sheet.

4. In a small bowl, mix together the olive oil, dried oregano, and garlic powder.

5. Brush the oil-herb mixture over the bell pepper halves, making sure to coat them evenly.

6. Season the peppers with salt and pepper to taste.

7. Roast the bell peppers for 20-25 minutes, or until they are tender and lightly charred.

8. Serve the roasted bell peppers warm or at room temperature.

Tips:
- Use low-sodium or no-salt-added seasonings to keep sodium content low.

- Avoid high-potassium ingredients like fresh herbs or balsamic vinegar.

- Adjust portion sizes as needed to fit individual dietary needs.

- This dish provides a good source of vitamins, minerals, and antioxidants.

This recipe for roasted bell peppers is a simple, flavorful side dish that is suitable for seniors with chronic kidney disease. The use of basic seasonings like oregano and garlic powder adds flavor without the need for high-sodium or high-potassium ingredients.

47. Rice pilaf

Ingredients:
- 1 cup uncooked white rice
- 1 tbsp olive oil
- 1/2 cup diced onion
- 1 tsp dried thyme
- 1/4 tsp garlic powder
- 2 cups low-sodium chicken or vegetable broth
- Salt and pepper to taste

Instructions:
1. In a medium saucepan, heat the olive oil over medium heat. Add the diced onion and sauté for 2-3 minutes, until translucent.

2. Add the uncooked white rice, dried thyme, and garlic powder. Stir to coat the rice with the oil and toast the grains for 1-2 minutes.

3. Pour in the low-sodium broth and bring the mixture to a boil.

4. Once boiling, reduce the heat to low, cover the saucepan, and simmer for 15-20 minutes, or until the rice is tender and the liquid is absorbed.

5. Remove the saucepan from the heat and let the rice pilaf rest, covered, for 5 minutes.

6. Fluff the rice pilaf with a fork and season with salt and pepper to taste. Serve the rice pilaf warm.

Tips:

- Use low-sodium or no-salt-added broth to keep sodium content low.

- Avoid high-potassium ingredients like mushrooms or peas.

- Adjust portion sizes as needed to fit individual dietary needs.

- This dish provides a good source of complex carbohydrates and can be a versatile base for other low-sodium, low-potassium dishes.

This simple rice pilaf recipe is a kidney-friendly option for seniors with chronic kidney disease. The use of basic seasonings and low-sodium broth helps to keep the sodium and potassium content in check.

48. Couscous with parsley

Ingredients:
- 1 cup uncooked pearl couscous
- 1 1/2 cups low-sodium chicken or vegetable broth
- 2 tbsp fresh parsley, chopped
- 1 tbsp olive oil
- 1/4 tsp garlic powder
- Salt and pepper to taste

Instructions:
1. In a medium saucepan, bring the low-sodium broth to a boil over high heat.

2. Once boiling, stir in the uncooked couscous, cover the saucepan, and remove it from the heat. Let the couscous sit for 5-7 minutes, or until the liquid is absorbed and the couscous is tender

3. Fluff the cooked couscous with a fork and transfer it to a serving bowl.

4. Stir in the chopped fresh parsley, olive oil, and garlic powder. Mix well to combine.

5. Season the couscous with salt and pepper to taste.

6. Serve the couscous with parsley warm or at room temperature.

Tips:
- Use low-sodium or no-salt-added broth to keep sodium content low.

- Avoid high-potassium herbs like cilantro or basil.

- Adjust portion sizes as needed to fit individual dietary needs.

- This dish provides a good source of complex carbohydrates and can be a versatile base for other low-sodium, low-potassium dishes.

This recipe for couscous with parsley is a simple, flavorful side dish that is suitable for seniors with chronic kidney disease. The use of low-sodium broth and the avoidance of high-potassium ingredients make it a kidney-friendly option.

49. Steamed carrots with honey glaze

Ingredients:
- 1 lb baby carrots, peeled and trimmed
- 1 tbsp olive oil
- 1 tbsp honey
- 1 tsp lemon juice
- 1/4 tsp ground cinnamon
- Salt and pepper to taste

Instructions:
1. Fill a large pot with 1-2 inches of water and bring it to a boil.

2. Place the peeled and trimmed baby carrots in a steamer basket and lower it into the pot. Cover and steam the carrots for 8-10 minutes, or until they are tender-crisp.

3. Drain the steamed carrots and transfer them to a serving bowl.

4. In a small bowl, whisk together the olive oil, honey, lemon juice, and ground cinnamon.

5. Drizzle the honey-cinnamon glaze over the steamed carrots and toss to coat them evenly.

6. Season the glazed carrots with salt and pepper to taste. Serve the steamed carrots with honey glaze warm.

Tips:

- Use low-sodium or no-salt-added seasonings to keep sodium content low.

- Avoid high-potassium ingredients like garlic or onions.

- Adjust portion sizes as needed to fit individual dietary needs.

- This dish provides a good source of vitamins, minerals, and natural sweetness from the honey.

This recipe for steamed carrots with a honey glaze is a simple, flavorful side dish that is suitable for seniors with chronic kidney disease. The use of honey and cinnamon adds sweetness without the need for high-sodium or high-potassium ingredients.

50. Garlic sautéed spinach

Ingredients:
- 1 lb fresh spinach, washed and stems removed
- 1 tbsp olive oil
- 2 cloves garlic, minced
- 1/4 tsp ground nutmeg
- Salt and pepper to taste

Instructions:
1. In a large skillet or wok, heat the olive oil over medium heat.

2. Add the minced garlic and sauté for 1 minute, until fragrant.

3. Working in batches if needed, add the fresh spinach to the skillet. Sauté the spinach, stirring frequently, until it is wilted and tender, about 3-5 minutes.

4. Remove the skillet from the heat and stir in the ground nutmeg.

5. Season the sautéed spinach with salt and pepper to taste.

6. Serve the garlic sautéed spinach warm.

Tips:
- Use low-sodium or no-salt-added seasonings to keep sodium content low.

- Avoid high-potassium ingredients like lemon juice or Parmesan cheese.

- Adjust portion sizes as needed to fit individual dietary needs.

- This dish provides a good source of vitamins, minerals, and antioxidants.

This recipe for garlic sautéed spinach is a simple, flavorful way to prepare this nutrient-dense vegetable that is suitable for seniors with chronic kidney disease. The use of garlic and nutmeg adds flavor without the need for high-sodium or high-potassium ingredients.

51. Unsalted popcorn

Ingredients:
- 1/2 cup unpopped popcorn kernels
- 1 tbsp olive oil or avocado oil

Instructions:
1. In a large pot with a tight-fitting lid, heat the oil over medium-high heat.

2. Add the unpopped popcorn kernels in a single layer and cover the pot.

3. Once the kernels start popping, shake the pot gently to prevent burning.

4. Continue shaking the pot until the popping slows to 2-3 seconds between pops.

5. Remove the pot from the heat and transfer the popped popcorn to a serving bowl.

6. Serve the unsalted popcorn warm.

Tips:
- Do not add any salt, butter, or other seasonings to the popcorn.

- Avoid high-potassium toppings like cheese or caramel.

- Adjust portion sizes as needed to fit individual dietary needs.

- This snack provides a good source of fiber and is low in sodium and potassium.

This recipe for unsalted popcorn is a simple, kidney-friendly snack option for seniors with chronic kidney disease. By avoiding added salt and high-potassium toppings, this popcorn can be enjoyed as a low-sodium, low-potassium treat.

52. Apple slices with peanut butter

Ingredients:
- 1 medium apple, cored and sliced into thin wedges
- 2 tbsp creamy peanut butter (look for a low-sodium variety)

Instructions:
1. Wash the apple and slice it into thin wedges, about 1/4 inch thick.

2. Spread 1-2 tsp of peanut butter onto each apple slice, using just enough to lightly coat the surface.

3. Arrange the apple slices with peanut butter on a plate and serve.

Tips for Seniors with Chronic Kidney Disease:

- Choose a low-potassium apple variety, such as Gala, Fuji or Honeycrisp.

- Limit peanut butter to 2 tbsp or less per serving to control phosphorus intake.

- Avoid adding any additional salt, as sodium intake should be restricted.

- Pair this snack with a small glass of water to stay hydrated.

- Monitor portion sizes, as both apples and peanut butter can be high in carbohydrates.

This simple snack provides a balance of carbohydrates, protein, and healthy fats to help support seniors with chronic kidney disease. The fiber from the apple and the protein/healthy fats from the peanut butter can also help promote feelings of fullness. As always, check with the healthcare team to ensure this snack fits the individual's dietary needs.

53. Carrot sticks with hummus

Ingredients:
- 2-3 medium carrots, peeled and cut into 4-inch sticks
- 2 tbsp low-sodium hummus

Instructions:
1. Wash and peel the carrots. Cut them into 4-inch sticks, about 1/2 inch thick.

2. Scoop 2 tbsp of low-sodium hummus into a small serving dish.

3. Arrange the carrot sticks around the hummus for dipping.

Tips for Seniors with Chronic Kidney Disease:

- Carrots are a great vegetable choice as they are low in potassium.

- Look for a hummus brand that is low in sodium, ideally less than 140mg per 2 tbsp serving.

- Limit the hummus portion to 2-3 tbsp to control phosphorus intake.

- Pair this snack with water to stay hydrated.

- Monitor portion sizes, as both carrots and hummus can contain carbohydrates.

- Check with the healthcare team to ensure this snack fits the individual's dietary needs.

This snack provides fiber, vitamins, and a source of plant-based protein from the hummus. The combination of crunchy carrots and creamy hummus can be satisfying for seniors. As always, portion control and sodium/phosphorus monitoring are important for those with chronic kidney disease.

54. Unsalted pretzels

Ingredients:
- Unsalted pretzels

Instructions:
1. Serve a small portion of unsalted pretzels, about 1-2 ounces (roughly 15-30 small pretzels).

Tips for Seniors with Chronic Kidney Disease:

- Pretzels are a good snack choice as they are low in potassium compared to many other salty snacks.

- Be sure to choose unsalted pretzels, as sodium intake needs to be limited with chronic kidney disease.

- Portion control is key, as pretzels can still contain carbohydrates that should be monitored.
- Pair the pretzels with a small glass of water to stay hydrated.

- Check with the healthcare team to ensure this snack fits the individual's dietary needs, as portion sizes may need to be adjusted.

Unsalted pretzels can provide a satisfying crunch and a source of carbohydrates for seniors with chronic kidney disease. The low potassium content makes them a better choice compared to many other salty snack options. As always, moderation and personalization based on the individual's health status are important.

55. Rice cakes with avocado

Ingredients:
- 2 plain, unsalted rice cakes
- 1/2 small avocado, mashed
- 1/4 tsp lemon juice (optional)
- Ground black pepper (optional)

Instructions:
1. Spread the mashed avocado evenly over the two rice cakes.

2. If desired, drizzle a small amount of lemon juice over the avocado and sprinkle with a pinch of ground black pepper.

Tips for Seniors with Chronic Kidney Disease:
- Rice cakes are a good low-potassium, low-sodium option for a snack base.

- Avocado is a healthy fat that can provide calories and nutrients without excessive potassium.

- Limit the amount of avocado to 1/2 small avocado or less to control phosphorus intake.

- Avoid adding any salt, as sodium intake should be restricted.

- The lemon juice can add a bit of flavor without additional sodium.

- Pair this snack with water to stay hydrated.

- Monitor portion sizes, as both rice cakes and avocado contain carbohydrates.

- Check with the healthcare team to ensure this snack fits the individual's dietary needs.

This simple snack provides a balance of complex carbohydrates, healthy fats, and a small amount of protein from the avocado. The combination of the crunchy rice cakes and creamy avocado can be satisfying for seniors with chronic kidney disease.

56. Fresh berries

Ingredients: 1 cup of fresh berries (such as blueberries, raspberries, or blackberries)

Instructions:
1. Rinse the fresh berries and place them in a small bowl.

Tips for Seniors with Chronic Kidney Disease:

- Berries are an excellent choice for seniors with chronic kidney disease as they are relatively low in potassium compared to many other fruits.

- Blueberries, raspberries, and blackberries are all good options.

- Portion control is important, as even low-potassium fruits should be limited to 1 cup or less per serving.

- Avoid adding any sugar or sweeteners, as these can increase the carbohydrate content.

- Pair the fresh berries with a small glass of water to stay hydrated.

- Check with the healthcare team to ensure the portion size and frequency of this snack fits the individual's dietary needs.

Fresh berries provide a sweet, refreshing snack that is high in antioxidants, fiber, and other beneficial nutrients. The low potassium content makes them a great choice for seniors with chronic kidney disease. As always, portion size and individual dietary requirements should be considered when incorporating this snack into the diet.

57. Celery sticks with cream cheese

Ingredients:
- 2-3 celery stalks, cut into 4-inch sticks
- 2 tbsp low-fat or reduced-fat cream cheese

Instructions:
1. Wash and cut the celery stalks into 4-inch sticks.

2. Spread 1-2 tsp of cream cheese onto each celery stick.

Tips for Seniors with Chronic Kidney Disease:

- Celery is a great vegetable choice as it is very low in potassium.

- Look for a cream cheese that is low in sodium, ideally less than 50mg per 2 tbsp serving.

- Limit the cream cheese portion to 2 tbsp or less to control phosphorus intake.

- Avoid adding any additional salt, as sodium intake should be restricted.

- Pair this snack with water to stay hydrated.

- Monitor portion sizes, as both celery and cream cheese can contain carbohydrates.

- Check with the healthcare team to ensure this snack fits the individual's dietary needs.

This simple snack provides a crunchy texture from the celery paired with the creamy, tangy flavor of the cream cheese. The combination can be satisfying for seniors. As always, portion control and monitoring of sodium and phosphorus intake are important for those with chronic kidney disease.

58. Low-sodium cheese cubes

Ingredients: 1 oz (about 1-2 small cubes) of low-sodium cheese, such as cheddar or Swiss

Instructions:
1. Cut a 1 oz portion of low-sodium cheese into small cubes.

Tips for Seniors with Chronic Kidney Disease:
- Cheese can be a good source of protein, but it is also high in sodium and phosphorus, which need to be limited with chronic kidney disease.

- Look for cheese varieties that are specifically labeled as "low-sodium" or "reduced-sodium." Aim for less than 140mg of sodium per 1 oz serving.

- Portion control is key - stick to a 1 oz serving (about 1-2 small cubes) to help manage phosphorus and sodium intake.

- Avoid pairing the cheese with high-sodium crackers or other salty accompaniments.

- Drink a small glass of water with this snack to stay hydrated.

- Check with the healthcare team to ensure this snack fits the individual's dietary needs, as portion sizes may need to be adjusted.

Low-sodium cheese cubes can provide a satisfying, protein-rich snack for seniors with chronic kidney disease when consumed in moderation. Careful selection of low-sodium varieties and appropriate portion sizes are important to meet dietary restrictions.

59. Unsweetened applesauce

Ingredients:
- 1/2 cup (4 oz) of unsweetened applesauce

Instructions:
1. Serve a 1/2 cup portion of unsweetened applesauce.

Tips for Seniors with Chronic Kidney Disease:

- Applesauce is a good low-potassium fruit option for those with chronic kidney disease.

- Be sure to choose an unsweetened variety, as added sugars can increase the carbohydrate content.

- Portion control is important, as even low-potassium fruits should be limited to 1/2 cup or less per serving.

- Avoid adding any additional sweeteners, as these can further increase the carbohydrate load.

- Pair the applesauce with a small glass of water to stay hydrated.

- Check with the healthcare team to ensure this snack fits the individual's dietary needs, as portion sizes may need to be adjusted.

Unsweetened applesauce can provide a smooth, lightly sweet snack option for seniors with chronic kidney disease. The low potassium content and lack of added sugars make it a better choice compared to many other fruit-based snacks. As always, portion control and personalization based on the individual's health status are important considerations.

60. Pear slices with honey

Ingredients:
- 1 small pear, cored and sliced
- 1 tsp honey

Instructions:
1. Wash and core the pear, then slice it into thin wedges.
2. Drizzle 1 tsp of honey over the pear slices.

Tips for Seniors with Chronic Kidney Disease:

- Pears are a good low-potassium fruit option for those with chronic kidney disease.

- Use only a small amount of honey, about 1 tsp, to provide a touch of sweetness without significantly increasing the carbohydrate content.

- Avoid adding any other sweeteners, as these can further increase the carbohydrate load.

- Portion control is important - limit the pear slices to 1 small pear or less per serving.

- Pair this snack with a small glass of water to stay hydrated.

- Check with the healthcare team to ensure this snack fits the individual's dietary needs, as portion sizes may need to be adjusted.

The combination of juicy pear slices and a light drizzle of honey can provide a refreshing, lightly sweet snack for seniors with chronic kidney disease. The low potassium content of pears makes them a better fruit choice, while the small amount of honey adds just a touch of sweetness without significantly impacting carbohydrate intake. As always, portion control and personalization based on the individual's health status are important considerations.

61. Berry sorbet

Ingredients:
- 1 cup frozen mixed berries (such as raspberries, blackberries, and blueberries)
- 2 tbsp water

Instructions:

1. In a food processor or high-powered blender, combine the frozen berries and water.

2. Blend until smooth and creamy, scraping down the sides as needed.

3. Serve the berry sorbet immediately.

Tips for Seniors with Chronic Kidney Disease:

- Berries are a good low-potassium fruit option for those with chronic kidney disease.

- The small amount of water helps blend the berries into a sorbet-like consistency without adding excess liquid.

- Avoid adding any sweeteners, as the natural sweetness of the berries should be sufficient.

- Portion control is important - limit the serving size to 1/2 cup or less.

- Serve the berry sorbet chilled for a refreshing, icy treat.

- Pair this snack with a small glass of water to stay hydrated.

- Check with the healthcare team to ensure this snack fits the individual's dietary needs, as portion sizes may need to be adjusted.

This simple berry sorbet provides a low-potassium, low-sodium frozen treat that can be a refreshing option for seniors with chronic kidney disease. The natural sweetness of the berries makes it a healthier alternative to traditional ice cream or sorbet.

62. Rice pudding with almond milk

Ingredients:
- 1/2 cup cooked white rice
- 1 cup unsweetened almond milk
- 1/2 tsp vanilla extract
- Ground cinnamon (optional)

Instructions:

1. In a small saucepan, combine the cooked white rice and unsweetened almond milk.

2. Heat the mixture over medium heat, stirring frequently, until it thickens to a pudding-like consistency, about 5-10 minutes.

3. Remove from heat and stir in the vanilla extract.

4. Serve warm, and if desired, sprinkle with a light dusting of ground cinnamon.

Tips for Seniors with Chronic Kidney Disease:

- White rice is a low-potassium grain option suitable for those with kidney disease.

- Unsweetened almond milk is low in potassium and phosphorus, making it a better choice than dairy milk.

- Avoid adding any sugar or other sweeteners, as these can increase the carbohydrate content.

- The vanilla extract provides a touch of flavor without additional nutrients of concern.

- Portion control is important - limit the serving size to 1/2 cup or less.

- Pair this snack with water to stay hydrated.

- Check with the healthcare team to ensure this recipe fits the individual's dietary needs.

This simple rice pudding made with almond milk can provide a comforting, lightly sweet snack for seniors with chronic kidney disease. The low-potassium ingredients make it a safer choice compared to traditional rice pudding recipes.

63. Low-sodium oatmeal cookies

Ingredients:
- 1 cup rolled oats
- 1/2 cup all-purpose flour
- 1/4 tsp baking powder
- 1/4 tsp ground cinnamon
- 1/4 cup unsalted butter, softened
- 1/4 cup brown sugar
- 1 egg
- 1 tsp vanilla extract

Instructions:
1. Preheat the oven to 350°F. Line a baking sheet with parchment paper.

2. In a medium bowl, combine the rolled oats, flour, baking powder, and cinnamon. Mix well.

3. In a separate bowl, cream the unsalted butter and brown sugar together until light and fluffy. Beat in the egg and vanilla extract.

4. Gradually add the dry ingredients to the wet ingredients, mixing until just combined. Scoop the dough by rounded tablespoons onto the prepared baking sheet, spacing them about 2 inches apart.

5. Bake for 10-12 minutes, or until the cookies are lightly golden. Allow the cookies to cool on the baking sheet for 5 minutes before transferring to a wire rack.

Tips for Seniors with Chronic Kidney Disease:

- Oatmeal is a good source of complex carbohydrates and fiber.

- Using unsalted butter and avoiding added salt helps keep the sodium content low.

- Portion control is important - limit to 1-2 cookies per serving.

- Avoid adding any additional toppings or mix-ins that may be high in sodium or potassium.

- Pair the cookies with a small glass of water to stay hydrated.

- Check with the healthcare team to ensure this snack fits the individual's dietary needs.

These low-sodium oatmeal cookies can provide a satisfying, lightly sweet treat for seniors with chronic kidney disease when consumed in moderation.

64. Apples baked with cinnamon

Ingredients:
- 2 medium apples, cored and sliced
- 1/2 tsp ground cinnamon
- 2 tbsp water

Instructions:

1. Preheat the oven to 375°F.

2. Core the apples and slice them into wedges, about 1/2 inch thick.

3. Arrange the apple slices in a baking dish and sprinkle with the ground cinnamon.

4. Pour the water into the baking dish, just enough to cover the bottom.

5. Bake for 20-25 minutes, or until the apples are tender and lightly caramelized.

6. Serve the baked apples warm.

Tips for Seniors with Chronic Kidney Disease:

- Apples are a good low-potassium fruit option for those with kidney disease.

- Cinnamon adds flavor without any additional sodium or potassium.

- Avoid adding any sweeteners, as the natural sweetness of the apples should be sufficient.

- Portion control is important - limit the serving size to 1 medium apple or less.

- Pair this snack with a small glass of water to stay hydrated.

- Check with the healthcare team to ensure this recipe fits the individual's dietary needs.

The baked apples with cinnamon provide a warm, comforting, and lightly sweet snack that is suitable for seniors with chronic kidney disease. The low-potassium content of the apples makes this a safer fruit option, while the cinnamon adds flavor without any additional nutrients of concern.

65. Lemon gelatin

Ingredients:
- 1 (3 oz) package of sugar-free, low-sodium lemon gelatin
- 1 cup unsweetened almond milk
- 1 cup water

Instructions:

1. In a medium saucepan, bring the 1 cup of water to a boil.

2. Remove the pan from heat and stir in the package of sugar-free, low-sodium lemon gelatin until completely dissolved.

3. Stir in the 1 cup of unsweetened almond milk.

4. Pour the gelatin mixture into individual serving dishes or a mold.

5. Refrigerate for at least 4 hours, or until set.

Tips for Seniors with Chronic Kidney Disease:
- Gelatin is a low-potassium, low-sodium dessert option.

- Using sugar-free, low-sodium gelatin helps control the carbohydrate and sodium content.

- Almond milk is a good alternative to dairy milk, as it is lower in potassium and phosphorus.

- Avoid adding any additional sweeteners, as the gelatin should provide enough sweetness.

- Portion control is important - limit the serving size to 1/2 cup or less.

- Serve the lemon gelatin chilled for a refreshing treat.

- Pair this snack with water to stay hydrated.

- Check with the healthcare team to ensure this recipe fits the individual's dietary needs.

This lemon gelatin made with almond milk can provide a light, refreshing snack option for seniors with chronic kidney disease. The low-potassium, low-sodium ingredients make it a safer choice compared to traditional gelatin desserts.

66. Peach crisp with oats

Filling Ingredients:
- 3 medium peaches, peeled, pitted, and sliced
- 1 tbsp all-purpose flour
- 1 tsp ground cinnamon

Topping Ingredients:
- 1/2 cup rolled oats
- 2 tbsp unsalted butter, softened
- 1 tbsp brown sugar
- 1/4 tsp ground cinnamon

Instructions:

1. Preheat the oven to 375°F. Grease a small baking dish.

2. In a bowl, toss the peach slices with the flour and 1 tsp of cinnamon. Spread the filling into the prepared baking dish.

3. In a separate bowl, mix together the rolled oats, softened butter, brown sugar, and 1/4 tsp cinnamon until well combined.

4. Sprinkle the oat topping evenly over the peach filling.

5. Bake for 20-25 minutes, or until the topping is lightly golden and the filling is bubbly.

6. Allow the crisp to cool for 5-10 minutes before serving.

Tips for Seniors with Chronic Kidney Disease:

- Peaches are a good low-potassium fruit option.

- Rolled oats provide a source of complex carbohydrates and fiber.

- Using unsalted butter and a small amount of brown sugar helps control sodium and phosphorus intake.

- Portion control is important - limit the serving size to 1/2 cup or less.

- Avoid adding any additional toppings or sweeteners.

- Pair this snack with a small glass of water to stay hydrated.

- Check with the healthcare team to ensure this recipe fits the individual's dietary needs.

This peach crisp with oats can provide a lightly sweet and comforting dessert-like snack for seniors with chronic kidney disease, while keeping the potassium, sodium, and phosphorus content in check.

67. Strawberry mousse

Ingredients:
- 1 cup fresh strawberries, hulled and sliced
- 1/4 cup granulated erythritol or other low-calorie sweetener
- 1 envelope (about 1 tbsp) unflavored gelatin
- 1 cup unsweetened almond milk
- 1 cup full-fat coconut milk
- 1 tsp vanilla extract

Instructions:

1. In a small saucepan, combine the sliced strawberries and erythritol. Cook over medium heat, stirring frequently, until the strawberries release their juices and the mixture is slightly thickened, about 5-7 minutes. Remove from heat and let cool slightly.

2. In a small bowl, sprinkle the gelatin over 2 tbsp of the almond milk. Let stand for 5 minutes to bloom.

3. In a medium saucepan, heat the remaining almond milk and the coconut milk over medium heat, stirring frequently, until steaming and bubbles start to form around the edges. Remove from heat.

4. Add the bloomed gelatin mixture to the warm milk mixture and whisk until the gelatin is completely dissolved.

5. Transfer the milk mixture to a blender. Add the cooked strawberries and vanilla extract. Blend until smooth and creamy.

6. Pour the strawberry mousse into individual serving dishes or ramekins. Refrigerate for at least 4 hours, or until set.

Tips for a PCOS-Friendly Fertility Diet:
- Strawberries are a low-glycemic fruit that can help manage blood sugar levels.

- Erythritol is a low-calorie sweetener that does not spike insulin levels.Gelatin can help support skin, hair, and nail health, which is important for fertility.

- Coconut milk provides healthy fats that are beneficial for hormone balance.Portion control is key - aim for 1/2 cup servings or less.

- Avoid added sugars, which can worsen PCOS symptoms.Pair the mousse with a small serving of nuts or seeds for additional protein and healthy fats

68. Blueberry compote

Ingredients:
- 2 cups fresh or frozen blueberries
- 2 tbsp granulated erythritol or other low-calorie sweetener
- 1 tbsp fresh lemon juice
- 1/4 tsp ground cinnamon

Instructions:
1. In a small saucepan, combine the blueberries, erythritol, lemon juice, and cinnamon.

2. Cook over medium heat, stirring occasionally, until the blueberries release their juices and the mixture thickens, about 10-15 minutes.

3. Remove from heat and let the compote cool slightly.

4. Serve the blueberry compote warm or chilled, over plain Greek yogurt, oatmeal, or as a topping for other PCOS-friendly desserts.

Tips for a PCOS-Friendly Fertility Diet:

- Blueberries are a low-glycemic fruit that are rich in antioxidants, which can help support fertility.

- Erythritol is a low-calorie sweetener that does not spike insulin levels, making it a better choice for those with PCOS.

- The lemon juice adds a touch of tartness and vitamin C, which is important for reproductive health.

- Cinnamon may help improve insulin sensitivity and reduce inflammation, both of which are beneficial for PCOS.

- Portion control is key - aim for 1/4 to 1/2 cup servings of the compote.

- Pair the compote with a source of protein, such as Greek yogurt, to help balance blood sugar levels.

- Avoid adding any additional sweeteners, as the erythritol and natural sweetness of the blueberries should be sufficient.

This blueberry compote can be a versatile and nutritious topping or accompaniment to various PCOS-friendly meals and snacks, supporting a fertility-focused diet.

69. Raspberry sherbet

Ingredients:
- 2 cups fresh or frozen raspberries
- 1/4 cup granulated erythritol or other low-calorie sweetener
- 1 cup unsweetened almond milk
- 1 tbsp fresh lemon juice

Instructions:
1. In a medium saucepan, combine the raspberries and erythritol. Cook over medium heat, stirring frequently, until the raspberries release their juices and the mixture is slightly thickened, about 5-7 minutes. Remove from heat and let cool slightly.

2. Transfer the raspberry mixture to a blender or food processor. Add the almond milk and lemon juice. Blend until smooth and creamy.

3. Pour the raspberry mixture into a shallow baking dish or freezer-safe container.

4. Freeze for 2 hours, then remove from the freezer and stir the mixture with a fork to break up any ice crystals.

5. Return the dish to the freezer and continue to freeze, stirring every 30 minutes, until the sherbet reaches your desired consistency, about 2-3 hours total.

6. Serve the raspberry sherbet immediately or transfer to an airtight container and freeze for up to 2 weeks.

Tips for a PCOS-Friendly Fertility Diet:
- Raspberries are a low-glycemic fruit that are rich in antioxidants, which can help support fertility.
- Erythritol is a low-calorie sweetener that does not spike insulin levels, making it a better choice for those with PCOS.
- Almond milk is a dairy-free option that is low in calories and carbohydrates.
- The lemon juice adds a touch of tartness and vitamin C, which is important for reproductive health.
- Portion control is key - aim for 1/2 cup servings or less of the sherbet.
- Avoid adding any additional sweeteners, as the erythritol and natural sweetness of the raspberries should be sufficient.
- Enjoy the raspberry sherbet as a refreshing and PCOS-friendly treat.

This raspberry sherbet can be a delightful and nutritious dessert option that supports a PCOS-friendly fertility diet for women.

70. Pineapple granita

Ingredients:
- 2 cups diced fresh pineapple
- 1/4 cup water
- 1 tbsp lime juice
- 1 tsp honey (optional)

Instructions:

1. In a blender, puree the diced pineapple, water, and lime juice until smooth.

2. Pour the pineapple mixture into a shallow baking dish or freezer-safe container.

3. Place the dish in the freezer and stir the mixture with a fork every 30 minutes, scraping the edges, until it reaches a granita-like, icy consistency, about 2-3 hours. If desired, drizzle the granita with 1 tsp of honey just before serving.

Tips for Seniors with Chronic Kidney Disease:

- Pineapple is a good low-potassium fruit option for those with kidney disease.

- The small amount of water and lime juice helps create the granita texture without adding excess liquid.

- The optional honey provides a touch of sweetness, but can be omitted if desired.

- Portion control is important - aim for 1/2 cup servings or less.

- Avoid adding any additional sweeteners, as the pineapple and honey (if used) should provide enough sweetness.

- Serve the pineapple granita chilled for a refreshing, icy treat.

- Pair this snack with a small glass of water to stay hydrated.

- Check with the healthcare team to ensure this recipe fits the individual's dietary needs.

This pineapple granita can be a light, refreshing, and low-potassium snack option for seniors with chronic kidney disease. The icy texture and natural sweetness of the pineapple make it a suitable and enjoyable treat.

71. Lemon water

Benefits of Lemon Water for Chronic Kidney Disease:
- Lemons are low in potassium, making them a safe fruit option for those with kidney disease.

- The citric acid in lemons can help increase citrate levels, which may help prevent kidney stone formation.

- Staying hydrated is crucial for kidney health, and lemon water can encourage increased fluid intake.

- Lemons contain vitamin C, which is an important antioxidant for overall health.

How to Make Lemon Water:
1. Fill a pitcher or water bottle with fresh, cool water.

2. Slice 1-2 lemons and add the slices to the water.

3. Allow the lemon slices to infuse the water for at least 30 minutes before drinking.

4. Refill the pitcher or bottle with more water as needed, reusing the lemon slices.

Tips for Seniors with Chronic Kidney Disease:
- Avoid adding any sweeteners, as these can increase the carbohydrate content.

- Limit the number of lemon slices to 1-2 per 8 oz glass of water to control the citric acid intake.

- Drink lemon water throughout the day to stay hydrated.

- Monitor fluid intake and check with the healthcare team on recommended daily fluid limits.

- Lemon water can be enjoyed chilled or at room temperature, depending on personal preference.

Lemon water is a simple, refreshing, and kidney-friendly beverage that can help support the overall health of seniors with chronic kidney disease when consumed in moderation.

72. Herbal teas (without added potassium)

1. Chamomile Tea:
  - Chamomile is a soothing, low-potassium herbal tea.
  - It can help promote relaxation and may have anti-inflammatory properties.

2. Peppermint Tea:
  - Peppermint tea is a refreshing, low-potassium option.
  - It may help with digestion and can provide a gentle energy boost.

3. Ginger Tea:
  - Ginger tea is low in potassium and can help settle the stomach.
  - It has anti-inflammatory properties and may improve circulation.

4. Rooibos Tea:
  - Rooibos, also known as red tea, is naturally caffeine-free and low in potassium.
  - It has a naturally sweet, earthy flavor and is rich in antioxidants.

5. Hibiscus Tea:
  - Hibiscus tea is low in potassium and has a tart, refreshing taste.
  - It may help support healthy blood pressure levels.

Tips for Seniors with Chronic Kidney Disease:

- Avoid herbal teas that are high in potassium, such as nettle, dandelion, or green tea.

- Steep the tea bags or loose leaf tea in hot water for 5-7 minutes to extract the full flavor.

- Drink the herbal teas plain, without adding any sweeteners, milk, or other ingredients.

- Limit intake to 1-2 cups per day and stay hydrated by pairing the tea with water.

- Check with the healthcare team to ensure the herbal teas fit within the individual's dietary needs.

These low-potassium herbal teas can provide a soothing, flavorful, and hydrating beverage option for seniors with chronic kidney disease.

73. Cranberry juice (in moderation)

1. Cranberry Smoothie:
   - 1 cup unsweetened cranberry juice
   - 1 cup low-fat plain Greek yogurt
   - 1 banana
   - 1 cup frozen mixed berries
   - Blend all ingredients until smooth.

2. Cranberry Spinach Salad:
   - 4 cups fresh spinach
   - 1/2 cup fresh cranberries
   - 2 tablespoons crumbled feta cheese
   - 2 tablespoons chopped walnuts
   - 2 tablespoons balsamic vinaigrette (made with a small amount of cranberry juice)

3. Cranberry Baked Chicken:
   - 4 boneless, skinless chicken breasts
   - 1/2 cup unsweetened cranberry juice
   - 2 tablespoons honey
   - 1 teaspoon dried thyme
   - Bake the chicken at 375°F for 25-30 minutes, basting with the cranberry-honey mixture.

4. Cranberry Oatmeal:
   - 1 cup cooked oatmeal
   - 1/4 cup unsweetened cranberry juice
   - 1 tablespoon chopped walnuts
   - 1 teaspoon honey (optional)

Remember to consult with a healthcare professional, as dietary needs may vary for individuals with chronic kidney disease. Moderation is key when it comes to cranberry juice, as it can be high in potassium and may interact with certain medications.

74. Apple juice (in moderation)

1. Apple Cinnamon Smoothie:
  - 1 cup unsweetened apple juice
  - 1 cup low-fat plain Greek yogurt
  - 1 banana
  - 1/2 teaspoon ground cinnamon
  - Blend all ingredients until smooth.

2. Apple Spinach Salad:
  - 4 cups fresh spinach
  - 1/2 cup diced apples
  - 2 tablespoons crumbled feta cheese
  - 2 tablespoons chopped walnuts
  - 2 tablespoons apple cider vinaigrette (made with a small amount of apple juice)

3. Baked Pork Chops with Apple Glaze:
  - 4 boneless pork chops
  - 1/2 cup unsweetened apple juice
  - 2 tablespoons honey
  - 1 teaspoon Dijon mustard
  - Bake the pork chops at 375°F for 25-30 minutes, basting with the apple-honey glaze.

4. Apple Cinnamon Oatmeal:
  - 1 cup cooked oatmeal
  - 1/4 cup unsweetened apple juice
  - 1 tablespoon chopped walnuts
  - 1 teaspoon honey (optional)
  - 1/4 teaspoon ground cinnamon

Remember to consult with a healthcare professional, as dietary needs may vary for individuals with chronic kidney disease. Moderation is key when it comes to apple juice, as it can be high in potassium and may interact with certain medications.

75. Rice milk

1. Rice Milk Smoothie:
  - 1 cup unsweetened rice milk
  - 1 banana
  - 1/2 cup frozen mixed berries
  - 1 tablespoon almond butter
  - Blend all ingredients until smooth.

2. Rice Milk Oatmeal:
  - 1 cup cooked oatmeal
  - 1/2 cup unsweetened rice milk
  - 1 tablespoon chopped walnuts
  - 1 teaspoon honey (optional)

3. Rice Milk Chia Pudding:
  - 1 cup unsweetened rice milk
  - 2 tablespoons chia seeds
  - 1 teaspoon vanilla extract
  - Mix all ingredients and let sit in the refrigerator for at least 2 hours, or overnight.

4. Rice Milk Custard:
  - 2 cups unsweetened rice milk
  - 2 eggs
  - 2 tablespoons honey
  - 1/2 teaspoon vanilla extract
  - Whisk all ingredients together and bake in a water bath at 325°F for 30-40 minutes, until set.

5. Rice Milk Mashed Potatoes:
  - 3 cups peeled and cubed potatoes
  - 1/2 cup unsweetened rice milk
  - 2 tablespoons butter
  - Salt and pepper to taste
  - Boil the potatoes, then mash with the rice milk and butter.

Remember to consult with a healthcare professional, as dietary needs may vary for individuals with chronic kidney disease. Rice milk can be a good alternative to cow's milk for those with kidney-related dietary restrictions.

76. Almond milk

1. Almond Milk Smoothie:
  - 1 cup unsweetened almond milk
  - 1 banana
  - 1/2 cup frozen berries
  - 1 tablespoon almond butter
  - Blend all ingredients until smooth.

2. Almond Milk Oatmeal:
  - 1 cup cooked oatmeal
  - 1/2 cup unsweetened almond milk
  - 1 tablespoon chopped almonds
  - 1 teaspoon honey (optional)

3. Almond Milk Chia Pudding:
  - 1 cup unsweetened almond milk
  - 2 tablespoons chia seeds
  - 1 teaspoon vanilla extract
  - Mix all ingredients and let sit in the refrigerator for at least 2 hours, or overnight.

4. Almond Milk Custard:
  - 2 cups unsweetened almond milk
  - 2 eggs
  - 2 tablespoons honey
  - 1/2 teaspoon vanilla extract
  - Whisk all ingredients together and bake in a water bath at 325°F for 30-40 minutes, until set.

5. Almond Milk Mashed Potatoes:
  - 3 cups peeled and cubed potatoes
  - 1/2 cup unsweetened almond milk
  - 2 tablespoons butter
  - Salt and pepper to taste
  - Boil the potatoes, then mash with the almond milk and butter.

Remember to consult with a healthcare professional, as dietary needs may vary for individuals with chronic kidney disease. Almond milk can be a good alternative to cow's milk for those with kidney-related dietary restrictions.

77. Unsweetened iced tea

1. Unsweetened Iced Tea Spritzer:
  - 1 cup unsweetened iced tea
  - 1/2 cup sparkling water
  - Lemon or lime wedge (optional)
  - Mix the iced tea and sparkling water, and garnish with a lemon or lime wedge.

2. Iced Tea and Fruit Salad:
  - 2 cups unsweetened iced tea, chilled
  - 1 cup diced fresh fruit (such as berries, melon, or pineapple)
  - 1 tablespoon chopped mint (optional)
  - Combine the iced tea, fruit, and mint (if using) in a bowl.

3. Iced Tea Popsicles:
  - 2 cups unsweetened iced tea, chilled
  - Lemon or lime slices (optional)
  - Pour the iced tea into popsicle molds and freeze until solid. You can add lemon or lime slices for extra flavor.

4. Iced Tea Lemonade:
  - 1 cup unsweetened iced tea
  - 1/2 cup freshly squeezed lemon juice
  - 1 cup water
  - Mix the iced tea, lemon juice, and water. Adjust to taste.

5. Iced Tea Smoothie:
  - 1 cup unsweetened iced tea, chilled
  - 1 banana
  - 1/2 cup frozen mixed berries
  - 1 tablespoon almond butter
  - Blend all ingredients until smooth.

Remember to consult with a healthcare professional, as dietary needs may vary for individuals with chronic kidney disease. Unsweetened iced tea can be a refreshing and hydrating option for seniors with kidney-related dietary restrictions.

78. Sparkling water with lime

1. Sparkling Lime Water:
   - 1 cup sparkling water
   - 1-2 lime wedges
   - Add the lime wedges to the sparkling water and enjoy.

2. Sparkling Lime Mocktail:
   - 1 cup sparkling water
   - 1/4 cup unsweetened cranberry juice
   - 1 lime wedge
   - Mix the sparkling water and cranberry juice, and garnish with a lime wedge.

3. Sparkling Lime Fruit Infusion:
   - 1 cup sparkling water
   - 1/2 cup diced watermelon or other low-potassium fruit
   - 1 lime wedge
   - Add the diced fruit and lime wedge to the sparkling water.

4. Sparkling Lime Iced Tea:
   - 1 cup unsweetened iced tea, chilled
   - 1/2 cup sparkling water
   - 1 lime wedge
   - Mix the iced tea and sparkling water, and garnish with a lime wedge.

5. Sparkling Lime Smoothie:
   - 1 cup sparkling water
   - 1 cup frozen low-potassium fruit (such as berries or melon)
   - 1 lime wedge
   - Blend the sparkling water, frozen fruit, and lime wedge until smooth.

Remember to consult with a healthcare professional, as dietary needs may vary for individuals with chronic kidney disease. Sparkling water with lime can be a refreshing and hydrating option for seniors with kidney-related dietary restrictions.

79. Blueberry smoothie with almond milk

Ingredients:
- 1 cup unsweetened almond milk
- 1 cup frozen blueberries
- 1 banana
- 1 tablespoon almond butter
- 1 teaspoon honey (optional)

Instructions:
1. Add all the ingredients to a blender.

2. Blend on high speed until the mixture is smooth and creamy.

3. Pour into a glass and enjoy.

Nutritional Benefits:

- Almond milk is low in potassium and a good alternative to dairy milk for those with chronic kidney disease.

- Blueberries are a good source of antioxidants and are relatively low in potassium.

- Bananas provide natural sweetness, but can be high in potassium, so they should be used in moderation.

- Almond butter adds healthy fats and protein without significantly increasing the potassium content.

- Honey can be used to add a touch of sweetness, if desired, but should also be used in moderation.

This smoothie can be a nutritious and refreshing option for seniors with chronic kidney disease, providing a balance of nutrients while keeping potassium levels in check. As always, it's important to consult with a healthcare professional to ensure this recipe fits within the individual's dietary needs.

80. Strawberry lemonade

Ingredients:
- 1 cup fresh or frozen strawberries
- 1/2 cup freshly squeezed lemon juice (about 3-4 lemons)
- 1/4 cup water
- 1-2 tablespoons honey (optional)
- Ice cubes

Instructions:
1. In a blender, puree the strawberries until smooth.

2. Strain the strawberry puree through a fine-mesh sieve to remove the seeds.

3. In a pitcher, combine the strained strawberry puree, lemon juice, and water. Stir well.

4. Taste and add honey if desired, to adjust sweetness.

5. Fill glasses with ice cubes and pour the strawberry lemonade over the top.

6. Garnish with a lemon slice or fresh strawberry, if desired.

Nutritional Benefits:

- Strawberries are a good source of vitamin C and relatively low in potassium, making them a suitable fruit for those with chronic kidney disease.

- Lemon juice is a good source of vitamin C and is low in potassium.

- Honey can be used to add sweetness, but should be used in moderation due to its high sugar content.

This strawberry lemonade can be a refreshing and hydrating option for seniors with chronic kidney disease. As always, it's important to consult with a healthcare professional to ensure this recipe fits within the individual's dietary needs.

81. Chicken salad with low-sodium dressing

Ingredients:
- 2 cups cooked, shredded chicken breast
- 1/2 cup diced celery
- 1/4 cup diced onion
- 1/4 cup diced apple
- 2 tablespoons chopped parsley
- 1/4 cup low-sodium mayonnaise
- 1 tablespoon lemon juice
- 1 teaspoon Dijon mustard
- 1/4 teaspoon ground black pepper

Instructions:

1. In a large bowl, combine the shredded chicken, celery, onion, apple, and parsley.

2. In a small bowl, whisk together the low-sodium mayonnaise, lemon juice, Dijon mustard, and black pepper.

3. Pour the dressing over the chicken salad and mix well to coat.

4. Serve the chicken salad on a bed of lettuce, or use it to make sandwiches or wraps.

Nutritional Benefits:

- Chicken is a lean protein source that is low in sodium and suitable for those with chronic kidney disease.

- Celery, onion, and apple provide fiber and vitamins without significantly increasing the potassium content.

- The low-sodium mayonnaise, lemon juice, and Dijon mustard create a flavorful dressing that is low in sodium.

This chicken salad can be a nutritious and satisfying option for seniors with chronic kidney disease. As always, it's important to consult with a healthcare professional to ensure this recipe fits within the individual's dietary needs.

82. Turkey and cranberry sandwich on whole wheat

Ingredients:
- 2 slices of whole wheat bread
- 3 ounces of sliced turkey breast
- 2 tablespoons of unsweetened cranberry sauce
- 1 tablespoon of low-sodium mayonnaise
- 1 leaf of lettuce (optional)

Instructions:
1. Spread the low-sodium mayonnaise on one slice of the whole wheat bread.

2. Layer the sliced turkey breast on top of the mayonnaise.

3. Spread the unsweetened cranberry sauce on the other slice of whole wheat bread.

4. Place the lettuce leaf (if using) on top of the cranberry sauce.

5. Carefully place the two slices of bread together to create the sandwich.

Nutritional Benefits:

- Whole wheat bread is a good source of fiber and complex carbohydrates, which can be beneficial for individuals with chronic kidney disease.

- Turkey breast is a lean protein source that is low in sodium and suitable for those with kidney-related dietary restrictions.

- Unsweetened cranberry sauce is a good source of antioxidants and is relatively low in potassium.

- The low-sodium mayonnaise helps to add moisture and flavor to the sandwich without significantly increasing the sodium content.

This turkey and cranberry sandwich on whole wheat bread can be a nutritious and satisfying option for seniors with chronic kidney disease. As always, it's important to consult with a healthcare professional to ensure this recipe fits within the individual's dietary needs.

83. Tuna salad with low-sodium mayo

Ingredients:
- 2 (5-ounce) cans of water-packed tuna, drained
- 2 tablespoons of low-sodium mayonnaise
- 1 tablespoon of diced celery
- 1 tablespoon of diced onion
- 1 teaspoon of lemon juice
- 1/4 teaspoon of ground black pepper

Instructions:

1. In a medium-sized bowl, combine the drained tuna, low-sodium mayonnaise, diced celery, diced onion, lemon juice, and ground black pepper.

2. Mix all the ingredients together until well combined.

3. Serve the tuna salad on a bed of lettuce, or use it to make sandwiches or wraps.

Nutritional Benefits:

- Tuna is a lean protein source that is low in sodium and suitable for those with chronic kidney disease.

- The low-sodium mayonnaise helps to add moisture and flavor to the tuna salad without significantly increasing the sodium content.

- Celery and onion provide some crunch and flavor without adding a significant amount of potassium.

- Lemon juice adds a refreshing tang without increasing the sodium content.

This tuna salad with low-sodium mayonnaise can be a nutritious and versatile option for seniors with chronic kidney disease. As always, it's important to consult with a healthcare professional to ensure this recipe fits within the individual's dietary needs.

84. Grilled vegetable wrap

Ingredients:
- 1 whole wheat tortilla or wrap
- 1/2 cup grilled or roasted vegetables (such as zucchini, bell peppers, onions, and mushrooms)
- 2 tablespoons of low-sodium hummus
- 1 tablespoon of crumbled feta cheese (optional)
- 1 leaf of lettuce (optional)

Instructions:
1. Grill or roast the vegetables until they are tender and slightly charred. Allow them to cool slightly.

2. Spread the low-sodium hummus evenly over the whole wheat tortilla or wrap.

3. Layer the grilled or roasted vegetables on top of the hummus.

4. If using, add the crumbled feta cheese and the lettuce leaf.

5. Carefully roll up the tortilla or wrap, ensuring that the filling is evenly distributed. Serve the grilled vegetable wrap immediately.

Nutritional Benefits:

- Whole wheat tortillas or wraps are a good source of fiber and complex carbohydrates, which can be beneficial for individuals with chronic kidney disease.

- Grilled or roasted vegetables are low in sodium and potassium, providing a variety of vitamins and minerals.

- Low-sodium hummus adds protein and healthy fats without significantly increasing the sodium content.

- Feta cheese is a low-sodium cheese option that can provide additional flavor and nutrients.

- Lettuce adds crunch and hydration without adding significant amounts of potassium.

This grilled vegetable wrap can be a nutritious and satisfying option for seniors with chronic kidney disease. As always, it's important to consult with a healthcare professional to ensure this recipe fits within the individual's dietary needs.

85. Egg salad sandwich

Ingredients:
- 4 hard-boiled eggs, peeled and chopped
- 2 tablespoons of low-sodium mayonnaise
- 1 teaspoon of Dijon mustard
- 1 tablespoon of diced celery
- 1 tablespoon of diced onion
- 1/4 teaspoon of ground black pepper
- 2 slices of whole wheat bread

Instructions:
1. In a medium-sized bowl, combine the chopped hard-boiled eggs, low-sodium mayonnaise, Dijon mustard, diced celery, diced onion, and ground black pepper.

2. Mix all the ingredients together until well combined.

3. Spread the egg salad mixture evenly on one slice of the whole wheat bread.

4. Top with the other slice of whole wheat bread to create the sandwich.

Nutritional Benefits:

- Eggs are a good source of protein and are low in sodium, making them a suitable option for those with chronic kidney disease.

- The low-sodium mayonnaise and Dijon mustard help to add flavor and moisture to the egg salad without significantly increasing the sodium content.

- Celery and onion provide some crunch and flavor without adding a significant amount of potassium.

- Whole wheat bread is a good source of fiber and complex carbohydrates, which can be beneficial for individuals with chronic kidney disease.

This egg salad sandwich can be a nutritious and satisfying option for seniors with chronic kidney disease. As always, it's important to consult with a healthcare professional to ensure this recipe fits within the individual's dietary needs.

86. Chicken and rice bowl

Ingredients:
- 1 cup cooked brown rice
- 4 ounces grilled or baked chicken breast, diced
- 1/2 cup diced bell peppers
- 1/4 cup diced onion
- 1 tablespoon low-sodium soy sauce or tamari
- 1 teaspoon sesame oil
- 1/4 teaspoon ground black pepper

Instructions:

1. Cook the brown rice according to package instructions.

2. In a medium bowl, combine the cooked brown rice, diced chicken, diced bell peppers, and diced onion.

3. In a small bowl, whisk together the low-sodium soy sauce or tamari, sesame oil, and ground black pepper.

4. Pour the dressing over the chicken and rice mixture and stir to coat evenly. Serve the chicken and rice bowl warm.

Nutritional Benefits:

- Brown rice is a good source of fiber and complex carbohydrates, which can be beneficial for individuals with chronic kidney disease.

- Chicken breast is a lean protein source that is low in sodium and suitable for those with kidney-related dietary restrictions.

- Bell peppers and onions provide a variety of vitamins and minerals without significantly increasing the potassium content.

- The low-sodium soy sauce or tamari and sesame oil add flavor without adding too much sodium.

This chicken and rice bowl can be a nutritious and satisfying option for seniors with chronic kidney disease. As always, it's important to consult with a healthcare professional to ensure this recipe fits within the individual's dietary needs.

87. Turkey and avocado sandwich

Ingredients:
- 2 slices of whole wheat bread
- 3 ounces of sliced turkey breast
- 1/2 of a ripe avocado, sliced
- 1 tablespoon of low-sodium mayonnaise
- 1 leaf of lettuce (optional)

Instructions:

1. Spread the low-sodium mayonnaise on one slice of the whole wheat bread.

2. Layer the sliced turkey breast on top of the mayonnaise.

3. Arrange the sliced avocado on top of the turkey.

4. If using, place the lettuce leaf on top of the avocado.

5. Place the other slice of whole wheat bread on top to complete the sandwich.

Nutritional Benefits:

- Whole wheat bread is a good source of fiber and complex carbohydrates, which can be beneficial for individuals with chronic kidney disease.

- Turkey breast is a lean protein source that is low in sodium and suitable for those with kidney-related dietary restrictions.

- Avocado is a good source of healthy fats and is relatively low in potassium, making it a suitable option for those with chronic kidney disease.

- The low-sodium mayonnaise helps to add moisture and flavor to the sandwich without significantly increasing the sodium content.

- Lettuce adds crunch and hydration without adding significant amounts of potassium.

This turkey and avocado sandwich can be a nutritious and satisfying option for seniors with chronic kidney disease. As always, it's important to consult with a healthcare professional to ensure this recipe fits within the individual's dietary needs.

88. Low-sodium ham and cheese sandwich

Ingredients:
- 2 slices of whole wheat bread
- 2 ounces of low-sodium ham
- 1 ounce of low-sodium cheddar cheese, sliced
- 1 tablespoon of low-sodium mayonnaise
- 1 leaf of lettuce (optional)

Instructions:
1. Spread the low-sodium mayonnaise on one slice of the whole wheat bread.

2. Layer the low-sodium ham on top of the mayonnaise.

3. Place the sliced low-sodium cheddar cheese on top of the ham.

4. If using, place the lettuce leaf on top of the cheese.

5. Place the other slice of whole wheat bread on top to complete the sandwich.

Nutritional Benefits:

- Whole wheat bread is a good source of fiber and complex carbohydrates, which can be beneficial for individuals with chronic kidney disease.

- Low-sodium ham is a good source of protein and is lower in sodium compared to regular ham, making it a suitable option for those with kidney-related dietary restrictions.

- Low-sodium cheddar cheese provides calcium and protein without significantly increasing the sodium content.

- The low-sodium mayonnaise helps to add moisture and flavor to the sandwich without significantly increasing the sodium content.

- Lettuce adds crunch and hydration without adding significant amounts of potassium.

This low-sodium ham and cheese sandwich can be a nutritious and satisfying option for seniors with chronic kidney disease. As always, it's important to consult with a healthcare professional to ensure this recipe fits within the individual's dietary needs.

89. Roasted chicken breast with quinoa

Ingredients:
- 4 ounces boneless, skinless chicken breast
- 1/2 cup cooked quinoa
- 1/2 cup diced bell peppers
- 1/4 cup diced onion
- 1 tablespoon olive oil
- 1 teaspoon dried thyme
- 1/4 teaspoon ground black pepper

Instructions:
1. Preheat your oven to 400°F (200°C).

2. Place the chicken breast on a baking sheet and drizzle with 1 teaspoon of olive oil. Season with 1/2 teaspoon of dried thyme and a pinch of black pepper.

3. Roast the chicken in the preheated oven for 20-25 minutes, or until the internal temperature reaches 165°F (75°C).

4. In a small bowl, combine the cooked quinoa, diced bell peppers, diced onion, the remaining 1/2 teaspoon of dried thyme, and the remaining 2 teaspoons of olive oil. Season with the remaining 1/4 teaspoon of black pepper.Serve the roasted chicken breast on top of the quinoa mixture.

Nutritional Benefits:

- Chicken breast is a lean protein source that is low in sodium and suitable for those with chronic kidney disease.

- Quinoa is a gluten-free grain that is high in protein, fiber, and various vitamins and minerals, making it a good choice for individuals with chronic kidney disease.

- Bell peppers and onions provide a variety of vitamins and minerals without significantly increasing the potassium content.

- Olive oil is a healthy source of monounsaturated fats. Dried thyme and black pepper add flavor without increasing the sodium content.

This roasted chicken breast with quinoa can be a nutritious and satisfying option for seniors with chronic kidney disease. As always, it's important to consult with a healthcare professional to ensure this recipe fits within the individual's dietary needs.

90. Tofu and vegetable stir-fry

Ingredients:
- 4 ounces firm or extra-firm tofu, cubed
- 1 cup mixed vegetables (such as broccoli, bell peppers, and snow peas)
- 1 tablespoon low-sodium soy sauce or tamari
- 1 teaspoon sesame oil
- 1 clove of garlic, minced
- 1/4 teaspoon ground ginger
- 1/4 teaspoon ground black pepper
- 1 cup cooked brown rice

Instructions:
1. In a large skillet or wok, heat the sesame oil over medium-high heat.

2. Add the minced garlic and sauté for 30 seconds, or until fragrant.

3. Add the cubed tofu and stir-fry for 2-3 minutes, until lightly browned.

4. Add the mixed vegetables and continue to stir-fry for 3-4 minutes, or until the vegetables are tender-crisp.

5. Stir in the low-sodium soy sauce or tamari, ground ginger, and black pepper. Toss to coat the tofu and vegetables evenly. Serve the tofu and vegetable stir-fry over the cooked brown rice.

Nutritional Benefits:
- Tofu is a good source of plant-based protein and is low in sodium, making it a suitable option for those with chronic kidney disease.

- The mixed vegetables provide a variety of vitamins, minerals, and fiber without significantly increasing the potassium content.

- Brown rice is a good source of complex carbohydrates and fiber, which can be beneficial for individuals with chronic kidney disease.

- The low-sodium soy sauce or tamari, sesame oil, garlic, and ginger add flavor without adding too much sodium.

This tofu and vegetable stir-fry can be a nutritious and flavorful option for seniors with chronic kidney disease. As always, it's important to consult with a healthcare professional to ensure this recipe fits within the individual's dietary needs.

91. Baked salmon with dill sauce

Ingredients:
- 4 ounces salmon fillet
- 1 tablespoon olive oil
- 1/4 teaspoon dried dill
- 1/4 teaspoon ground black pepper

Dill Sauce:
- 2 tablespoons low-fat plain Greek yogurt
- 1 teaspoon lemon juice
- 1 teaspoon chopped fresh dill (or 1/2 teaspoon dried dill)
- 1/8 teaspoon garlic powder
- 1/8 teaspoon ground black pepper

Instructions:
1. Preheat your oven to 400°F (200°C).

2. Place the salmon fillet on a baking sheet lined with parchment paper. Drizzle with the olive oil and sprinkle with the dried dill and black pepper.

3. Bake the salmon in the preheated oven for 12-15 minutes, or until it flakes easily with a fork.

4. In a small bowl, mix together the ingredients for the dill sauce: Greek yogurt, lemon juice, fresh or dried dill, garlic powder, and black pepper.

5. Serve the baked salmon warm, with the dill sauce on the side.

Nutritional Benefits:
- Salmon is a good source of omega-3 fatty acids, which can be beneficial for individuals with chronic kidney disease.

- The dill sauce provides a flavorful topping without significantly increasing the sodium content.

- Greek yogurt is a good source of protein and is lower in sodium compared to regular yogurt. Lemon juice and garlic powder add flavor without adding sodium.

This baked salmon with dill sauce can be a nutritious and delicious option for seniors with chronic kidney disease. As always, it's important to consult with a healthcare professional to ensure this recipe fits within the individual's dietary needs.

92. Grilled turkey cutlets with herbs

Ingredients:
- 4 ounces turkey cutlets
- 1 tablespoon olive oil
- 1 teaspoon dried thyme
- 1 teaspoon dried rosemary
- 1/4 teaspoon ground black pepper

Instructions:
1. Preheat your grill or grill pan to medium-high heat.

2. In a small bowl, mix together the olive oil, dried thyme, dried rosemary, and black pepper.

3. Brush the turkey cutlets with the herb mixture, coating both sides evenly.

4. Grill the turkey cutlets for 3-4 minutes per side, or until they are cooked through and reach an internal temperature of 165°F (75°C).

5. Serve the grilled turkey cutlets warm.

Nutritional Benefits:

- Turkey is a lean protein source that is low in sodium and suitable for those with chronic kidney disease.

- The herbs, such as thyme and rosemary, add flavor without increasing the sodium content.
- Olive oil is a healthy source of monounsaturated fats.

- Black pepper adds flavor without adding sodium.

This grilled turkey cutlets with herbs recipe can be a nutritious and flavorful option for seniors with chronic kidney disease. The lean protein from the turkey, combined with the herbs and spices, can make for a satisfying and kidney-friendly meal.

As always, it's important to consult with a healthcare professional to ensure this recipe fits within the individual's dietary needs and restrictions.

93. Pork chops with apple compote

Ingredients:
- 4 ounces boneless pork chops
- 1 tablespoon olive oil
- 1/2 cup unsweetened applesauce
- 1 tablespoon lemon juice
- 1/4 teaspoon ground cinnamon
- 1/8 teaspoon ground nutmeg
- 1/4 teaspoon ground black pepper

Instructions:
1. Preheat your oven to 400°F (200°C).

2. Heat the olive oil in a large oven-safe skillet over medium-high heat.

3. Season the pork chops with the black pepper and add them to the hot skillet. Sear the pork chops for 2-3 minutes per side, or until they are lightly browned.

4. Transfer the skillet to the preheated oven and bake the pork chops for 10-12 minutes, or until they reach an internal temperature of 145°F (63°C).

5. In a small bowl, mix together the unsweetened applesauce, lemon juice, cinnamon, and nutmeg to make the apple compote. Serve the pork chops warm, topped with the apple compote.

Nutritional Benefits:

- Pork chops are a good source of protein and are relatively low in sodium, making them a suitable option for those with chronic kidney disease.

- Unsweetened applesauce is a good source of fiber and is low in potassium, making it a suitable fruit option for individuals with kidney-related dietary restrictions.

- Lemon juice, cinnamon, and nutmeg add flavor without increasing the sodium content.

This pork chops with apple compote recipe can be a nutritious and flavorful option for seniors with chronic kidney disease. The combination of the lean pork and the low-potassium apple compote can make for a satisfying and kidney-friendly meal.

As always, it's important to consult with a healthcare professional to ensure this recipe fits within the individual's dietary needs and restrictions.

94. Chicken and broccoli casserole

Ingredients:
- 4 ounces boneless, skinless chicken breast, diced
- 1 cup chopped broccoli florets
- 1/2 cup cooked brown rice
- 1/4 cup low-sodium chicken broth
- 2 tablespoons low-fat plain Greek yogurt
- 1 tablespoon grated Parmesan cheese
- 1/4 teaspoon dried thyme
- 1/4 teaspoon ground black pepper

Instructions:

1. Preheat your oven to 375°F (190°C).

2. In a medium-sized bowl, combine the diced chicken, chopped broccoli, cooked brown rice, low-sodium chicken broth, Greek yogurt, Parmesan cheese, dried thyme, and black pepper. Mix well to ensure all the ingredients are evenly distributed.

3. Transfer the mixture to a small baking dish or casserole dish.

4. Bake the casserole in the preheated oven for 25-30 minutes, or until the chicken is cooked through and the broccoli is tender. Serve the chicken and broccoli casserole warm.

Nutritional Benefits:

- Chicken breast is a lean protein source that is low in sodium and suitable for those with chronic kidney disease.

- Broccoli is a low-potassium vegetable that provides fiber, vitamins, and minerals.

- Brown rice is a good source of complex carbohydrates and fiber, which can be beneficial for individuals with chronic kidney disease.

- The low-sodium chicken broth and low-fat Greek yogurt help to add moisture and creaminess to the casserole without significantly increasing the sodium content.

- Parmesan cheese and dried thyme add flavor without adding too much sodium.

This chicken and broccoli casserole can be a nutritious and comforting option for seniors with chronic kidney disease. As always, it's important to consult with a healthcare professional to ensure this recipe fits within the individual's dietary needs and restrictions.

95. Baked cod with garlic and herbs

Ingredients:
- 4 ounces cod fillet
- 1 tablespoon olive oil
- 1 clove of garlic, minced
- 1 teaspoon dried parsley
- 1/2 teaspoon dried thyme
- 1/4 teaspoon ground black pepper

Instructions:
1. Preheat your oven to 400°F (200°C).

2. Place the cod fillet in a baking dish or on a parchment-lined baking sheet.

3. In a small bowl, mix together the olive oil, minced garlic, dried parsley, dried thyme, and black pepper.

4. Spread the garlic and herb mixture evenly over the top of the cod fillet.

5. Bake the cod in the preheated oven for 15-18 minutes, or until the fish flakes easily with a fork and reaches an internal temperature of 145°F (63°C).

6. Serve the baked cod warm.

Nutritional Benefits:

- Cod is a lean, low-sodium fish that is a good source of protein, making it a suitable option for those with chronic kidney disease.

- Olive oil is a healthy source of monounsaturated fats.

- Garlic, parsley, and thyme add flavor without increasing the sodium content.

- Black pepper provides a subtle seasoning without adding sodium.

This baked cod with garlic and herbs recipe can be a nutritious and flavorful option for seniors with chronic kidney disease. The combination of the lean protein from the cod and the herbs and spices can make for a satisfying and kidney-friendly meal.

As always, it's important to consult with a healthcare professional to ensure this recipe fits within the individual's dietary needs and restrictions.

96. Beef and vegetable kebabs

Ingredients:
- 4 ounces beef sirloin, cut into 1-inch cubes
- 1 cup chopped vegetables (such as bell peppers, zucchini, and onions)
- 1 tablespoon olive oil
- 1 teaspoon dried oregano
- 1/4 teaspoon ground black pepper

Instructions:
1. Preheat your grill or grill pan to medium-high heat.

2. In a medium bowl, combine the beef cubes, chopped vegetables, olive oil, dried oregano, and black pepper. Toss to coat the ingredients evenly.

3. Thread the beef and vegetables onto skewers, alternating the ingredients.

4. Grill the kebabs for 8-10 minutes, turning occasionally, until the beef is cooked through and the vegetables are tender.

5. Serve the beef and vegetable kebabs warm.

Nutritional Benefits:

- Beef sirloin is a lean protein source that is relatively low in sodium, making it a suitable option for those with chronic kidney disease.

- The vegetables, such as bell peppers, zucchini, and onions, are low in potassium and provide a variety of vitamins and minerals.

- Olive oil is a healthy source of monounsaturated fats.

- Dried oregano adds flavor without increasing the sodium content.

- Black pepper provides a subtle seasoning without adding sodium.

This beef and vegetable kebab recipe can be a nutritious and flavorful option for seniors with chronic kidney disease. The combination of the lean protein from the beef and the low-potassium vegetables can make for a satisfying and kidney-friendly meal.

As always, it's important to consult with a healthcare professional to ensure this recipe fits within the individual's dietary needs and restrictions.

97. Stuffed bell peppers with rice

Ingredients:
- 2 medium bell peppers, halved and seeded
- 1/2 cup cooked brown rice
- 2 ounces ground turkey or chicken
- 1/4 cup diced onion
- 1 clove of garlic, minced
- 1 tablespoon low-sodium tomato sauce
- 1/4 teaspoon dried oregano
- 1/4 teaspoon ground black pepper
- 1 tablespoon grated low-sodium cheese (optional)

Instructions:
1. Preheat your oven to 375°F (190°C).

2. Place the bell pepper halves in a baking dish or on a parchment-lined baking sheet.

3. In a medium bowl, mix together the cooked brown rice, ground turkey or chicken, diced onion, minced garlic, low-sodium tomato sauce, dried oregano, and black pepper.

4. Spoon the rice and meat mixture evenly into the bell pepper halves.

5. If using, sprinkle the grated low-sodium cheese over the top of the stuffed peppers.

6. Bake the stuffed bell peppers in the preheated oven for 25-30 minutes, or until the peppers are tender and the filling is heated through. Serve the stuffed bell peppers warm.

Nutritional Benefits:
- Bell peppers are a low-potassium vegetable that provides fiber, vitamins, and minerals.

- Brown rice is a good source of complex carbohydrates and fiber, which can be beneficial for individuals with chronic kidney disease. Ground turkey or chicken is a lean protein source that is low in sodium.

- The low-sodium tomato sauce and grated low-sodium cheese (if used) add flavor without significantly increasing the sodium content. Onion and garlic provide additional flavor without adding too much sodium.

This stuffed bell pepper with rice recipe can be a nutritious and satisfying option for seniors with chronic kidney disease. As always, it's important to consult with a healthcare professional to ensure this recipe fits within the individual's dietary needs and restrictions.

98. Lemon garlic shrimp

Ingredients:
- 4 ounces raw shrimp, peeled and deveined
- 1 tablespoon olive oil
- 2 cloves of garlic, minced
- 1 tablespoon lemon juice
- 1/4 teaspoon dried parsley
- 1/4 teaspoon ground black pepper

Instructions:
1. In a medium skillet, heat the olive oil over medium heat.

2. Add the minced garlic to the hot oil and sauté for 1 minute, or until fragrant.

3. Add the raw shrimp to the skillet and cook for 2-3 minutes per side, or until the shrimp are opaque and cooked through.

4. Remove the skillet from the heat and stir in the lemon juice, dried parsley, and black pepper.

5. Serve the lemon garlic shrimp warm, over a bed of steamed vegetables or a small portion of cooked brown rice.

Nutritional Benefits:
- Shrimp is a lean protein source that is low in sodium and suitable for those with chronic kidney disease.

- Olive oil is a healthy source of monounsaturated fats.

- Garlic and lemon juice add flavor without increasing the sodium content.

- Dried parsley provides a subtle herb flavor without adding sodium.

- Black pepper adds seasoning without increasing the sodium content.

This lemon garlic shrimp recipe can be a nutritious and flavorful option for seniors with chronic kidney disease. The combination of the lean protein from the shrimp and the low-sodium seasonings can make for a satisfying and kidney-friendly meal.

As always, it's important to consult with a healthcare professional to ensure this recipe fits within the individual's dietary needs and restrictions.

99. Chicken thighs with rosemary and thyme

Ingredients:
- 4 ounces boneless, skinless chicken thighs
- 1 tablespoon olive oil
- 1 teaspoon dried rosemary
- 1 teaspoon dried thyme
- 1/4 teaspoon ground black pepper

Instructions:
1. Preheat your oven to 400°F (200°C).

2. Place the chicken thighs in a baking dish or on a parchment-lined baking sheet.

3. Drizzle the olive oil over the chicken thighs and rub it in to coat them evenly.

4. Sprinkle the dried rosemary, dried thyme, and black pepper over the chicken thighs, making sure to distribute the seasonings evenly.

5. Bake the chicken thighs in the preheated oven for 25-30 minutes, or until they reach an internal temperature of 165°F (75°C).

6. Serve the chicken thighs warm.

Nutritional Benefits:

- Chicken thighs are a good source of protein and are relatively low in sodium, making them a suitable option for those with chronic kidney disease.

- Olive oil is a healthy source of monounsaturated fats.

- Dried rosemary and thyme add flavor without increasing the sodium content.

- Black pepper provides a subtle seasoning without adding sodium.

This chicken thighs with rosemary and thyme recipe can be a nutritious and flavorful option for seniors with chronic kidney disease. The combination of the lean protein from the chicken and the herbs can make for a satisfying and kidney-friendly meal.

As always, it's important to consult with a healthcare professional to ensure this recipe fits within the individual's dietary needs and restrictions.

100. Herb-roasted chicken

Ingredients:
- 1 whole chicken, cut into 8 pieces (or use 4 ounces of chicken thighs and drumsticks)
- 1 tablespoon olive oil
- 1 teaspoon dried thyme
- 1 teaspoon dried rosemary
- 1/4 teaspoon ground black pepper

Instructions:
1. Preheat your oven to 400°F (200°C).

2. Place the chicken pieces in a large baking dish or on a parchment-lined baking sheet.

3. Drizzle the olive oil over the chicken and rub it in to coat the pieces evenly.

4. Sprinkle the dried thyme, dried rosemary, and black pepper over the chicken, making sure to distribute the seasonings evenly.

5. Roast the chicken in the preheated oven for 35-40 minutes, or until the chicken is cooked through and the juices run clear.

6. Serve the herb-roasted chicken warm.

Nutritional Benefits:

- Chicken is a lean protein source that is relatively low in sodium, making it a suitable option for those with chronic kidney disease.

- Olive oil is a healthy source of monounsaturated fats.

- Dried thyme and rosemary add flavor without increasing the sodium content.

- Black pepper provides a subtle seasoning without adding sodium.

This herb-roasted chicken recipe can be a nutritious and flavorful option for seniors with chronic kidney disease. The combination of the lean protein from the chicken and the herbs can make for a satisfying and kidney-friendly meal.

As always, it's important to consult with a healthcare professional to ensure this recipe fits within the individual's dietary needs and restrictions.

101. Lentil stew

Ingredients:
- 1/2 cup dry brown or green lentils, rinsed
- 2 cups low-sodium vegetable broth
- 1 cup diced carrots
- 1/2 cup diced celery
- 1/2 cup diced onion
- 2 cloves of garlic, minced
- 1 teaspoon dried thyme
- 1/4 teaspoon ground black pepper
- 1 tablespoon lemon juice (optional)

Instructions:
1. In a medium saucepan, combine the rinsed lentils and low-sodium vegetable broth. Bring the mixture to a boil over high heat.

2. Once boiling, reduce the heat to low, cover the saucepan, and simmer for 15-20 minutes, or until the lentils are tender.

3. Add the diced carrots, celery, onion, and minced garlic to the saucepan. Continue to simmer for an additional 10-15 minutes, or until the vegetables are tender.

4. Stir in the dried thyme and black pepper. Taste and adjust seasoning as needed.

5. If desired, stir in the lemon juice just before serving. Serve the lentil stew warm.

Nutritional Benefits:
- Lentils are a good source of plant-based protein, fiber, and various vitamins and minerals, making them a suitable ingredient for those with chronic kidney disease.

- Carrots, celery, and onion provide additional nutrients without significantly increasing the potassium content.

- The low-sodium vegetable broth helps to keep the sodium content in check.

- Dried thyme and black pepper add flavor without increasing the sodium content.Lemon juice can provide a refreshing touch of acidity, if desired.

This lentil stew can be a nutritious and comforting option for seniors with chronic kidney disease. As always, it's important to consult with a healthcare professional to ensure this recipe fits within the individual's dietary needs and restrictions.

102. Quinoa and black bean stuffed peppers

Ingredients:
- 2 medium bell peppers, halved and seeded
- 1/2 cup cooked quinoa
- 1/2 cup canned low-sodium black beans, rinsed and drained
- 1/4 cup diced onion
- 1 clove of garlic, minced
- 1 tablespoon low-sodium salsa
- 1/4 teaspoon ground cumin
- 1/4 teaspoon dried oregano
- 1/8 teaspoon ground black pepper

Instructions:
1. Preheat your oven to 375°F (190°C).

2. Place the bell pepper halves in a baking dish or on a parchment-lined baking sheet.

3. In a medium bowl, combine the cooked quinoa, black beans, diced onion, minced garlic, low-sodium salsa, cumin, dried oregano, and black pepper. Mix well. Spoon the quinoa and black bean mixture evenly into the bell pepper halves.

4. Bake the stuffed peppers in the preheated oven for 25-30 minutes, or until the peppers are tender and the filling is heated through. Serve the quinoa and black bean stuffed peppers warm.

Nutritional Benefits:
- Bell peppers are a low-potassium vegetable that provides fiber, vitamins, and minerals.

- Quinoa is a gluten-free grain that is high in protein, fiber, and various nutrients, making it a suitable option for those with chronic kidney disease.

- Canned low-sodium black beans are a good source of plant-based protein and fiber. Onion and garlic provide additional flavor without adding too much sodium.

- The low-sodium salsa, cumin, and oregano add flavor without significantly increasing the sodium content.

This quinoa and black bean stuffed pepper recipe can be a nutritious and satisfying option for seniors with chronic kidney disease. As always, it's important to consult with a healthcare professional to ensure this recipe fits within the individual's dietary needs and restrictions.

103. Tofu stir-fry with mixed vegetables

Ingredients:
- 4 ounces firm or extra-firm tofu, cubed
- 1 tablespoon low-sodium soy sauce or tamari
- 1 teaspoon sesame oil
- 1 cup mixed vegetables (such as broccoli, bell peppers, and snow peas), chopped
- 1 clove of garlic, minced
- 1 teaspoon grated fresh ginger
- 1/4 teaspoon ground black pepper
- 1 cup cooked brown rice

Instructions:
1. In a medium bowl, toss the cubed tofu with the low-sodium soy sauce or tamari and sesame oil. Set aside.

2. In a large skillet or wok, stir-fry the mixed vegetables, minced garlic, and grated ginger over medium-high heat for 3-4 minutes, or until the vegetables are tender-crisp.

3. Add the marinated tofu to the skillet and continue to stir-fry for an additional 2-3 minutes, until the tofu is heated through.

4. Season the stir-fry with the ground black pepper. Serve the tofu and vegetable stir-fry over the cooked brown rice.

Nutritional Benefits:

- Tofu is a good source of plant-based protein and is low in sodium, making it a suitable option for those with chronic kidney disease.

- The mixed vegetables, such as broccoli, bell peppers, and snow peas, provide a variety of vitamins, minerals, and fiber without significantly increasing the potassium content.

- Brown rice is a good source of complex carbohydrates and fiber, which can be beneficial for individuals with chronic kidney disease.

- The low-sodium soy sauce or tamari, sesame oil, garlic, and ginger add flavor without adding too much sodium.

This tofu stir-fry with mixed vegetables can be a nutritious and flavorful option for seniors with chronic kidney disease. As always, it's important to consult with a healthcare professional to ensure this recipe fits within the individual's dietary needs and restrictions.

104. Spaghetti squash with marinara sauce

Ingredients:
- 1 medium spaghetti squash
- 1 tbsp olive oil
- 1 jar (24 oz) marinara sauce
- 1/4 cup grated Parmesan cheese (optional)
- Fresh basil, chopped (optional)

Instructions:

1. Preheat oven to 400°F. Cut the spaghetti squash in half lengthwise and scoop out the seeds. Place the squash halves cut-side up on a baking sheet. Drizzle with olive oil and season with salt and pepper.

2. Roast the spaghetti squash for 40-50 minutes, until tender when pierced with a fork. Allow to cool slightly.

3. Use a fork to scrape the flesh of the squash, separating it into spaghetti-like strands. Transfer the squash strands to a serving bowl.

4. Heat the marinara sauce in a saucepan over medium heat until warmed through.

5. Pour the warm marinara sauce over the spaghetti squash strands and toss to coat evenly.

6. Top with grated Parmesan cheese and fresh chopped basil, if desired.

7. Serve immediately and enjoy your healthy, low-carb spaghetti squash with marinara!

105. Chickpea salad

Ingredients:
- 1 (15 oz) can low-sodium chickpeas, rinsed and drained
- 1/4 cup diced celery
- 1/4 cup diced red onion
- 2 tbsp chopped fresh parsley
- 2 tbsp olive oil
- 1 tbsp lemon juice
- 1/4 tsp garlic powder
- 1/4 tsp ground black pepper
- 1/8 tsp salt (or to taste)

Instructions:

1. In a medium bowl, combine the rinsed and drained chickpeas, diced celery, diced red onion, and chopped parsley.

2. In a small bowl, whisk together the olive oil, lemon juice, garlic powder, black pepper, and salt.

3. Pour the dressing over the chickpea mixture and stir gently to coat everything evenly.

4. Taste and adjust seasoning as needed, adding more lemon juice, pepper, or a pinch of salt if desired.

5. Serve the chickpea salad chilled or at room temperature. It can be enjoyed on its own, on top of a bed of greens, or with whole grain crackers.

This recipe is kidney-friendly as it is low in sodium and phosphorus, two nutrients that need to be limited for those with chronic kidney disease. The chickpeas provide plant-based protein, fiber, and other beneficial nutrients. Enjoy this easy, flavorful salad as a healthy lunch or side dish.

106. Vegetable curry with rice

Ingredients:
- 1 cup uncooked basmati rice
- 1 tbsp olive oil
- 1 onion, diced
- 3 cloves garlic, minced
- 1 tbsp grated fresh ginger
- 1 tsp ground cumin
- 1 tsp ground coriander
- 1/2 tsp ground turmeric
- 1/4 tsp cayenne pepper (optional)
- 1 cup low-sodium vegetable broth
- 1 (15 oz) can low-sodium diced tomatoes
- 1 (15 oz) can low-sodium chickpeas, rinsed and drained
- 2 cups chopped cauliflower florets
- 1 cup chopped zucchini
- 1/4 cup chopped fresh cilantro
- Salt and pepper to taste

Instructions:

1. Cook the basmati rice according to package instructions. Set aside.

2. In a large skillet, heat the olive oil over medium heat. Add the diced onion and sauté for 5 minutes until translucent.

3. Add the minced garlic, grated ginger, cumin, coriander, turmeric, and cayenne (if using). Cook for 1 minute, stirring constantly, until fragrant.

4. Pour in the vegetable broth and diced tomatoes. Bring to a simmer.

5. Add the rinsed and drained chickpeas, cauliflower florets, and zucchini. Simmer for 10-15 minutes, until the vegetables are tender.

6. Stir in the chopped cilantro and season with salt and pepper to taste.

7. Serve the vegetable curry over the cooked basmati rice.

This curry is low in sodium, phosphorus, and potassium, making it kidney-friendly for those with chronic kidney disease. The vegetables, chickpeas, and rice provide a balanced, nutritious meal. Adjust spices to your taste preferences.

107. Grilled portobello mushrooms

Ingredients:
- 4 large portobello mushroom caps, stems removed
- 2 tbsp olive oil
- 1 tbsp balsamic vinegar
- 2 cloves garlic, minced
- 1 tsp dried thyme
- 1/4 tsp ground black pepper
- 1/8 tsp salt (or to taste)

Instructions:

1. Preheat grill or grill pan to medium-high heat.

2. In a shallow dish, whisk together the olive oil, balsamic vinegar, minced garlic, dried thyme, black pepper, and salt.

3. Add the portobello mushroom caps to the dish and turn to coat both sides evenly with the marinade.

4. Grill the mushrooms for 4-5 minutes per side, until tender and lightly charred.

5. Transfer the grilled portobello caps to a serving plate.

6. Optionally, you can top the mushrooms with a small amount of low-sodium feta cheese or chopped fresh herbs like parsley or basil.

Serve the grilled portobello mushrooms as a main dish, side, or as part of a larger meal. They pair well with roasted vegetables, quinoa, or a simple salad.

This recipe is kidney-friendly as it is low in sodium, phosphorus, and potassium - three nutrients that need to be limited for those with chronic kidney disease. The portobello mushrooms provide a meaty, satisfying texture and are a good source of antioxidants.

108. Bean and vegetable soup

Ingredients:
- 1 tbsp olive oil
- 1 onion, diced
- 2 carrots, peeled and diced
- 2 stalks celery, diced
- 3 cloves garlic, minced
- 1 tsp dried thyme
- 1/2 tsp dried oregano
- 1/4 tsp ground black pepper
- 4 cups low-sodium vegetable broth
- 1 (15 oz) can low-sodium white beans, rinsed and drained
- 1 (15 oz) can low-sodium kidney beans, rinsed and drained
- 2 cups chopped kale or spinach
- 1/4 cup chopped fresh parsley
- Salt to taste (optional)

Instructions:

1. In a large pot or Dutch oven, heat the olive oil over medium heat. Add the diced onion, carrots, and celery. Sauté for 5-7 minutes until the vegetables are softened.

2. Add the minced garlic, dried thyme, oregano, and black pepper. Cook for 1 minute, stirring constantly, until fragrant.

3. Pour in the low-sodium vegetable broth and bring the mixture to a simmer.

4. Add the rinsed and drained white beans and kidney beans. Simmer for 10 minutes.

5. Stir in the chopped kale or spinach and cook for 5 more minutes, until the greens are wilted.

6. Remove from heat and stir in the chopped fresh parsley.

7. Taste and add a small amount of salt if needed, keeping in mind the sodium restrictions for chronic kidney disease.

Serve the bean and vegetable soup hot. This recipe is kidney-friendly as it is low in sodium, phosphorus, and potassium. The beans provide plant-based protein, while the vegetables add fiber, vitamins, and minerals.

109. Vegetable and quinoa pilaf

Ingredients:
- 1 cup uncooked quinoa, rinsed
- 2 cups low-sodium vegetable broth
- 1 tbsp olive oil
- 1 onion, diced
- 2 carrots, peeled and diced
- 1 red bell pepper, diced
- 2 cloves garlic, minced
- 1 tsp ground cumin
- 1/2 tsp dried thyme
- 1/4 tsp ground black pepper
- 1/8 tsp salt (or to taste)
- 1 cup frozen peas
- 2 tbsp chopped fresh parsley

Instructions:

1. In a medium saucepan, combine the rinsed quinoa and vegetable broth. Bring to a boil, then reduce heat to low, cover, and simmer for 15-20 minutes, until the quinoa is tender and the liquid is absorbed. Fluff with a fork and set aside.

2. In a large skillet, heat the olive oil over medium heat. Add the diced onion, carrots, and bell pepper. Sauté for 5-7 minutes, until the vegetables are softened.

3. Stir in the minced garlic, cumin, thyme, black pepper, and salt (if using). Cook for 1 minute, until fragrant.

4. Add the cooked quinoa and frozen peas to the skillet. Stir to combine everything evenly.

5. Remove from heat and stir in the chopped fresh parsley.

6. Serve the vegetable and quinoa pilaf warm.

This pilaf is kidney-friendly as it is low in sodium, phosphorus, and potassium. The quinoa provides a good source of plant-based protein, while the vegetables add fiber, vitamins, and minerals. Adjust seasoning to your taste preferences.

110. Zucchini noodles with tomato basil sauce

Ingredients:
- 3 medium zucchini, spiralized or julienned into noodles
- 1 tbsp olive oil
- 3 cloves garlic, minced
- 1 (14 oz) can low-sodium diced tomatoes
- 1/4 cup chopped fresh basil
- 1/4 tsp ground black pepper
- 1/8 tsp salt (or to taste)
- 2 tbsp grated Parmesan cheese (optional)

Instructions:

1. Using a spiralizer or julienne peeler, cut the zucchini into long, thin noodles. Set aside.

2. In a large skillet, heat the olive oil over medium heat. Add the minced garlic and sauté for 1 minute, until fragrant.

3. Pour in the can of low-sodium diced tomatoes and their juices. Bring the mixture to a simmer.

4. Add the zucchini noodles to the skillet and toss to coat with the tomato sauce. Cook for 3-5 minutes, until the zucchini noodles are tender but still have a bit of bite.

5. Remove from heat and stir in the chopped fresh basil, black pepper, and salt (if using).

6. Serve the zucchini noodles with tomato basil sauce immediately. Top with a sprinkle of grated Parmesan cheese, if desired.

This recipe is kidney-friendly as it is low in sodium, phosphorus, and potassium. The zucchini noodles provide a low-carb, low-calorie alternative to traditional pasta. The tomato-basil sauce is full of flavor without being overly salty.

Adjust the salt to your taste preferences, keeping in mind the sodium restrictions for those with chronic kidney disease. Enjoy this healthy, veggie-packed meal!

111. Mango sorbet

Ingredients:
- 2 cups diced fresh mango (or frozen mango, thawed)
- 1/4 cup water
- 2 tbsp lime juice
- 1 tbsp honey (or maple syrup)
- 1/8 tsp salt

Instructions:

1. In a blender or food processor, combine the diced mango, water, lime juice, honey, and salt. Blend until smooth and creamy.

2. Pour the mango mixture into a shallow baking dish or metal pan. Cover and freeze for 2 hours, stirring and scraping the sides every 30 minutes, until partially frozen.

3. Once partially frozen, transfer the mixture to a blender or food processor and blend again until smooth and creamy. This helps create a smooth, sorbet-like texture.

4. Return the blended mango mixture to the baking dish or pan and freeze for an additional 2-3 hours, stirring and scraping the sides every 30 minutes, until completely frozen.

5. Scoop the mango sorbet into serving dishes and enjoy immediately.

This mango sorbet is a refreshing and kidney-friendly dessert. It is low in sodium, phosphorus, and potassium - three nutrients that need to be limited for those with chronic kidney disease.

The mango provides natural sweetness, while the lime juice and honey (or maple syrup) add a touch of tartness and balance the flavors. The small amount of salt helps enhance the overall taste.

Feel free to adjust the sweetener to your personal taste preferences. Enjoy this delicious and nutritious mango sorbet!

112. Banana bread with low-sodium baking powder

Ingredients:
- 1 1/2 cups all-purpose flour
- 1 tsp low-sodium baking powder
- 1/2 tsp baking soda
- 1/4 tsp ground cinnamon
- 1/8 tsp salt
- 3 ripe bananas, mashed (about 1 cup)
- 1/2 cup granulated sugar
- 1/4 cup unsweetened applesauce
- 2 tbsp vegetable oil
- 1 egg
- 1 tsp vanilla extract

Instructions:

1. Preheat your oven to 350°F. Grease a 9x5-inch loaf pan with non-stick cooking spray.

2. In a medium bowl, whisk together the all-purpose flour, low-sodium baking powder, baking soda, cinnamon, and salt. Set aside.

3. In a large bowl, mash the ripe bananas until smooth. Add the granulated sugar, unsweetened applesauce, vegetable oil, egg, and vanilla extract. Stir until well combined.

4. Gradually add the dry ingredients from the medium bowl to the wet ingredients, mixing just until incorporated. Do not overmix.

5. Pour the banana bread batter into the prepared loaf pan, smoothing the top.

6. Bake for 55-65 minutes, or until a toothpick inserted in the center comes out clean.

7. Allow the banana bread to cool in the pan for 10 minutes, then transfer to a wire rack to cool completely before slicing.

This banana bread recipe is kidney-friendly as it uses low-sodium baking powder, which helps reduce the overall sodium content. The bananas provide natural sweetness, while the applesauce and oil keep the bread moist without adding too much fat.

Enjoy this delicious and nutritious banana bread as a snack or breakfast for seniors with chronic kidney disease.

113. Cinnamon apple chips

Ingredients:
- 2 medium apples, cored and thinly sliced (about 1/8-inch thick)
- 1 tsp ground cinnamon
- 1/8 tsp ground nutmeg (optional)

Instructions:

1. Preheat your oven to 200°F. Line two baking sheets with parchment paper or silicone baking mats.

2. Arrange the apple slices in a single layer on the prepared baking sheets. Make sure the slices are not overlapping.

3. Sprinkle the apple slices evenly with the ground cinnamon and nutmeg (if using).

4. Bake for 1 to 1 1/2 hours, flipping the apple slices halfway through, until they are crisp and dried out.

5. Turn off the oven and leave the apple chips inside for an additional 1 to 2 hours, or until they have reached your desired crispness.

6. Remove the apple chips from the oven and let them cool completely on the baking sheets.

7. Once cooled, transfer the cinnamon apple chips to an airtight container for storage.

These cinnamon apple chips are a healthy, kidney-friendly snack for seniors with chronic kidney disease. They are low in sodium, phosphorus, and potassium, making them a great option.

The natural sweetness of the apples and the warm spices of cinnamon and nutmeg create a delicious flavor. These chips can be enjoyed on their own or as a topping for yogurt or oatmeal.

Store the apple chips in an airtight container at room temperature for up to 1 week.

114. Strawberry banana smoothie

Ingredients:
- 1 cup frozen strawberries
- 1 medium ripe banana, frozen
- 1 cup unsweetened almond milk
- 1 tbsp honey (or maple syrup)
- 1/2 tsp vanilla extract
- 1/8 tsp ground cinnamon (optional)

Instructions:

1. In a high-speed blender, combine the frozen strawberries, frozen banana, unsweetened almond milk, honey (or maple syrup), and vanilla extract.

2. Blend on high speed until the mixture is smooth and creamy, about 1-2 minutes.

3. If desired, add a pinch of ground cinnamon and blend again briefly to incorporate.

4. Pour the strawberry banana smoothie into a glass and serve immediately.

This smoothie is kidney-friendly for seniors with chronic kidney disease for a few reasons:

1. It's low in sodium, phosphorus, and potassium - three nutrients that need to be limited for those with CKD.

2. The almond milk is a good dairy-free alternative that is also low in these key minerals.

3. The fruit provides natural sweetness without added sugars.

4. The honey (or maple syrup) adds a touch of sweetness while being a better option than table sugar.

Feel free to adjust the amount of honey/maple syrup to your taste preferences. You can also add a handful of spinach or kale for an extra nutrient boost.

Enjoy this refreshing and kidney-friendly strawberry banana smoothie as a healthy snack or light meal.

115. Pineapple slices with mint

Ingredients:
- 1 fresh pineapple, peeled, cored, and sliced into 1/2-inch thick rounds
- 2-3 tbsp fresh mint leaves, chopped

Instructions:

1. Arrange the pineapple slices on a serving platter or plate.

2. Sprinkle the chopped fresh mint leaves evenly over the pineapple slices.

3. Serve immediately or chill in the refrigerator until ready to serve.

This pineapple and mint combination makes for a light, refreshing, and kidney-friendly snack or dessert. Here's why it's suitable for seniors with chronic kidney disease:

- Pineapple is a good source of vitamin C and manganese, without being high in potassium or phosphorus.

- Fresh mint is low in sodium, potassium, and phosphorus, making it a great flavor enhancer.

- The dish does not contain any added sugars, salts, or other ingredients that may be problematic for those with kidney disease.

The natural sweetness of the pineapple pairs beautifully with the bright, cooling flavor of the mint. This simple preparation allows the fresh flavors to shine.

You can serve the pineapple slices chilled or at room temperature. They make a refreshing snack or light dessert, especially on a warm day.

Adjust the amount of mint to your personal taste preferences. Enjoy this kidney-friendly pineapple and mint treat!

*As you come to the end of the **Cookbook for Seniors: 110+ Recipes for Senior Adults Living with Chronic Kidney Disease,** we hope you feel equipped with the knowledge and inspiration to embrace a healthier and more flavorful approach to cooking and eating with CKD.*

Managing chronic kidney disease can present its challenges, but with the right tools and resources, it is possible to enjoy delicious and nourishing meals that support kidney health and overall well-being. This cookbook has been carefully curated with seniors in mind, offering a wide variety of recipes that are not only kidney-friendly but also satisfying to the senses.

Throughout these pages, you've discovered a wealth of recipes spanning breakfast, lunch, dinner, and snacks, each crafted with wholesome ingredients and thoughtful consideration for the nutritional needs of seniors with CKD. From hearty soups and comforting casseroles to vibrant salads and flavorful main courses, these recipes are sure to delight your taste buds while supporting your health goals.

But this cookbook is more than just a collection of recipes. It's a testament to the power of food as medicine and the importance of nourishing both body and soul. Each recipe is accompanied by valuable tips and insights, empowering you to make informed choices about your diet and lifestyle.

As you continue your journey with chronic kidney disease, remember that you are not alone. Whether you're cooking for yourself or a loved one, this cookbook is here to guide and support you every step of the way. Embrace the joy of cooking, savor the flavors of wholesome ingredients, and nourish yourself from the inside out.

Thank you for allowing this cookbook to be a part of your culinary adventure. Here's to good health, good food, and good living for seniors with chronic kidney disease. Cheers to your well-being and vitality!